Scholarship of Teaching and Learning in Speech-Language Pathology and Audiology

EVIDENCE-BASED EDUCATION

Scholarship of Teaching and Learning in Speech-Language Pathology and Audiology

EVIDENCE-BASED EDUCATION

Sarah M. Ginsberg, EdD
Jennifer C. Friberg, EdD
Colleen F. Visconti, PhD

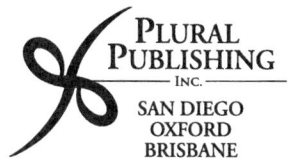

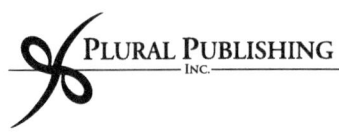

5521 Ruffin Road
San Diego, CA 92123

e-mail: information@pluralpublishing.com
Web site: https://www.pluralpublishing.com

Copyright © by Plural Publishing, Inc. 2012

Typeset in 10½/13 Palatino by Flanagan's Publishing Services, Inc.
Printed in the United States of America by McNaughton and Gunn
22 21 20 19   2 3 4 5

Cover artwork by Molly E. Friberg

All rights, including that of translation, reserved. No part of this publication may be reproduced, stored in a retrieval system, or transmitted in any form or by any means, electronic, mechanical, recording, or otherwise, including photocopying, recording, taping, Web distribution, or information storage and retrieval systems without the prior written consent of the publisher.

For permission to use material from this text, contact us by
Telephone: (866) 758-7251
Fax: (888) 758-7255
e-mail: permissions@pluralpublishing.com

Every attempt has been made to contact the copyright holders for material originally printed in another source. If any have been inadvertently overlooked, the publishers will gladly make the necessary arrangements at the first opportunity.

Library of Congress Cataloging-in-Publication Data:
Ginsberg, Sarah, 1966-
  Scholarship of teaching and learning in speech-language pathology and audiology : evidence-based education / Sarah Ginsberg, Jennifer Friberg, and Colleen F. Visconti.
     p. ; cm.
  Includes bibliographical references and index.
  ISBN-13: 978-1-59756-429-8 (alk. paper)
  ISBN-10: 1-59756-429-X (alk. paper)
  I. Friberg, Jennifer, 1974- II. Visconti, Colleen F., 1963- III. Title.
  [DNLM: 1. Speech Therapy--education. 2. Teaching--methods. 3. Audiology—education. 4. Evidence-Based Practice. 5. Language Therapy—education. 6. Learning. WL 340.3]
  LC-classification not assigned
  616.85'50071—dc23
                              2011028487

Contents

Foreword by L. Dee Fink, PhD .... *ix*
Foreword by Elizabeth McCrea, PhD .... *xiii*

1 Good Teaching, Scholarly Teaching, and Scholarship of Teaching ... 1
Fundamental Scholarship of Teaching and Learning Concepts ... 1
Dual Professions ... 3
Professional Educator Continuing Education ... 7
A Framework of Educator Development ... 9
Developing as Professional Educators: Working Toward Each Level ... 11

2 EBP in Clinical Practice versus EBE in Classroom Teaching ... 25
Evidence-Based Practice as the Foundation for Clinical Service Delivery ... 25
Evidence-Based Education as the Foundation for Classroom Teaching ... 28
Linking the Levels of Evidence in EBP to EBE ... 34
Why Do We Need EBE? ... 36
Where Do I Find the Evidence? ... 38
Now What Do I Do? ... 38

3 The "Learner Centered-Active Learning" Paradigm ... 41
Bloom's Taxonomy ... 42
Learner-Centered Instruction ... 47
Concluding Thoughts ... 53

4 Before You Teach: Course Design and Preparation   57
Backward Design   58
Evidence for Backward Design   64
Applying Backward Design: A Practice Example   65
Creating Significant Learning   65
Evidence for Creating Significant Learning   85
Application of Fink's Creating Significant Learning   88
Concluding Remarks   92

5 Communication in the Classroom   97
Instructional Communication Competence   98
Immediacy and Clarity   100
Teacher Transparency   111
Social Presence   114

6 Engaging the Learner   127
Collaborative Learning Techniques   128
Problem-Based Learning   137
Academic Service Learning   142
Technology for Engaged Learning   148

7 Assessing Student Learning   169
Overview of Assessment   170
Assessment Approaches   171
Tools for Assessment   182

8 Moving Forward Toward SOTL   197
Why We Need to Support Good, Scholarly Teaching and SOTL   197
Mechanisms of Support for Professional Development Toward SOTL   202
Teachers Researching Teaching: Action Research for SOTL   211
Ethical Considerations and SOTL   217
Dissemination of SOTL Work   226

⑨ SOTL as Part of Your Research Agenda   **237**
Planning Your SOTL Research Agenda   239
The Value of SOTL on Your Campus?   242
What Can Be Done?   245
Final Thoughts   248

Index   *251*

Foreword

By L. Dee Fink, PhD

This is a very important book. In fact, I wish every college professor would read it and just substitute the name of his or her discipline wherever "communication science" occurs. The perspectives and principles that Ginsberg, Friberg, and Visconti lay out here are universal; only the particulars are discipline-specific.

Let me explain why I think it is so important for all college teachers to understand the need for and how to engage in the Scholarship of Teaching and Learning, in the form of a three-level argument.

I. The Need for Change in Higher Education

Thomas Friedman, in his very influential book, *"The World is Flat"* (2005), described how information technology has changed the world in multiple ways. Two of those changes that have major significance for higher education are the rate and nature of change. As most of us can observe, changes are happening faster and faster. But, in addition, information technology has connected all parts of the world, and this means that both the opportunities and problems that we face are more multifaceted and complex.

This has two implications for higher education. First, as Friedman argues in his book: The flatter the world gets, the more *important* tertiary education becomes. And the world is only going to get flatter. And second, as others have also argued, the *kind* of education needed now is different than in the past. People need to know how to solve new kinds of problems. This means graduates need to know how to describe and structure new kinds of problems, how to identify and find relevant information, and then how to use that information. And all of this needs to happen in the context of small group work because that is how complex problems are and will be handled.

Unfortunately, there is lots of information that indicates American higher education is not educating its students well, even by traditionally valued kinds of learning. One of the most persuasive of these sources is the book by Derek Bok, former president of Harvard, who carefully examined the research evidence about how well graduates are achieving eight kinds of learning (e.g., communication skills, critical thinking, preparing for citizenship, living with diversity, preparing for a global society, etc.). In all eight areas, his conclusions were the same: students are achieving some of these goals, but at nowhere near the level that they *could* be and *should* be. Hence, the name of his book: *Our Underachieving Colleges: A Candid Look at How Much Our Students Learn and Why They Should Be Learning More* (2006).

II. What Changes Do We Need to Make?

If college teaching is very important but we are not doing as good a job as we should, what should we do differently?

We need to start by taking a new perspective on what we are doing as teachers. As Barr and Tagg argued in their classic article in 1995, we need to shift from a "Teaching Paradigm" to a "Learning Paradigm" of our work. When we take a teaching-centered view of our work, as most people do, we tend to see the standards of high quality work as: (a) Do I know a lot about the subject I teach? and (b) Do I communicate my knowledge in a well-organized way with some enthusiasm?

When we take a learning-centered view, the standards change to: (a) Did a large proportion of the students learn something important? and (b) Did they learn that *because of* my teaching (rather than *in spite of* it)? In this view, teaching is still important but now it is no longer the end itself but a means to a more important end. The real "bottom line" is the quality and quantity of student learning.

A second view that we need to accept, if we are going to change the overall quality of higher education, is that all of us, even the best among us, need to work at getting better—every year, every year.

III. The Value of Engaging in SoTL

If we accept the perspective of learning-centered teaching and the need for universal, continuous improvement, what are the action implications of that? This means we need to continuously learn about and learn how to use new ideas about teaching and learning. That is, this generation of teachers needs to create a way of teaching that is different from the way they were taught.

That is a big challenge, and this means we will need to help each other do it. And this means we need to share our experiences about what happens when we learn about, use, and assess the results of new ideas on teaching and learning. It will not suffice for professors to create a special experience and then hide the results "under a basket." We all need to share what we learn.

This Book

And that is what this book calls all professors to do: Engage in the practice of the Scholarship of Teaching and Learning (SoTL). This book provides a carefully organized introduction to SoTL and identifies multiple resources that will be very helpful when we engage in this process.

We need to break down the isolation that currently dominates our work as teachers, and share what we learn as we grow in our ability to generate high quality learning experiences for our students. If we can do that, our morale as teachers will go up and our ability to create high quality learning experiences will be greatly increased. And when that happens, the level of student engagement and the quantity and quality of student learning will also rise—the dream of every college teacher who *cares*!

We all owe a deep measure of appreciation to the authors for putting together such an importance resource for such an important task!

> L. Dee Fink, PhD
> Former President, POD Network in
>   Higher Education (2004–2005)
> Currently, an international consultant
>   in higher education and head of
>   Dee Fink & Associates

References

Barr, R. B. & Tagg, J. (1995). From teaching to learning: A new paradigm for undergraduate education. *Change Magazine, 27*(6), 13–25.

Bok, D. (2006). *Our underachieving colleges: A candid look at how much students learn and why they should be learning more.* Princeton, NJ: Princeton University Press.

Friedman, T. (2005). *The world is flat: A brief history of the twenty-first century.* New York, NY: Farrar, Straus, and Giroux.

Foreword

By Elizabeth McCrea, PhD

Members of the academic and clinical education communities in Communication Sciences and Disorders (CSD) undoubtedly consider one of their primary responsibilities to be the instruction and education of students in the basic science of the discipline and the theoretical constructs of disordered communication. In their very thoughtful book, the authors challenge us to apply the principles embedded in the Scholarship of Teaching and Learning (SOTL) to move our teaching from good teaching to professional teaching and ultimately, to scholarly teaching. The authors challenge us to think of ourselves as not just simply audiologists, speech-language pathologists, or speech-language-hearing scientists but as professional educators as well.

As students are asked to employ Evidence-Based Practice in their work with their patients and clients, the authors make the case that the scientific and scholarly bases for instruction by professional educators in the classroom contributes to the ability of students to develop the habits of mind, the analytical and cognitive behaviors, as well as the affective capacity, to sustain successful professional lives. Most educators would agree that there is no one way to teach, no one pedagogy that is appropriate in every didactic or clinical training situation; however, understanding which teaching approach or strategy produces the desired knowledge and/or skill outcome in a specific situation is the challenge for every educator.

To help educators adapt to different needs of students in different aspects of the curriculum, the authors develop the notions of Learner-Centered Instruction and Backward Design. In addition they provide resources and applied examples of each construct to support the reader in pursuit of these strategies in their own curricular design and student engagement. To complete this pedagogical discussion, the authors suggest multiple ways to assess student learning which are consistent with both Learner-Centered Instruction and Backward Design. These assessment strategies will also facilitate the ability of the educator to understand not only how successful the student has been in achieving learning outcomes but also how well the instruction has engaged students and addressed their diverse learning needs. The *Scholarship of Teaching and Learning in Speech-Language Pathology and Audiology: Evidence Based Education* concludes by emphasizing the importance of contributing to and participating in a SOTL community of professional and scholarly educators who actively reflect on their teaching; read and apply literature on teaching and learning; and most importantly, share their findings about teaching and learning in the discipline.

The authors have written a book that is logically sequenced and well-written. It is relatable and immensely easy to read and comprehend. It will be important to the library of every faculty person, irrespective of whether they are at the beginning or in the middle of their career. It is the first of its kind in Communication Sciences and Disorders and is a substantive contribution to the literature that grounds scholarly pedagogical activity in the academy. As such, it is important to the continued development of the academy and ultimately, to the students we teach.

Elizabeth McCrea, PhD, CCC-SLP
Clinical Professor Emerita
Indiana University

Dedication

*For all of our current and future colleagues,
and the students we all teach.*

*For our own children, Molly, Drew, Shannon, Bridget,
Claire, James, Jess and Max, the students of tomorrow.*

1

Good Teaching, Scholarly Teaching, and Scholarship of Teaching

> *Research begins in wonder and curiosity but ends in teaching*
> —Lee Shulman (www.leeshulman.net)

Fundamental Scholarship of Teaching and Learning Concepts

A little known fact among those engaged in the scholarship of teaching and learning (SOTL) is that the movement actually was started by an audiologist. In 1990, Ernest Boyer, then president of the Carnegie Foundation for the Advancement of Teaching (1975–1995) and a former audiology faculty member, wrote *Scholarship Reconsidered*, a text that broke new ground for academia. In this seminal text, Boyer argued that university faculty engaged in four different types of scholarship. Boyer called what we traditionally consider to be research within our discipline the "scholarship of discovery" (1990, p. 17). This research is based in the researcher's discipline and represents the uncovering of new, previously unknown, or not-understood material and is the heart of many academic institutions.

Boyer went on to describe the "scholarship of integration" (p. 18), which aims to make connections between bodies of knowledge. By engaging in the scholarship of integration, we draw information from within our own disciplines as well as finding relationships to knowledge that comes from a variety of fields. The scholarship of integration is, as Boyer noted, closely related to the scholarship of discovery, as any time that we discover something, we must determine how our newly uncovered knowledge integrates with what was known before and how it extends our knowledge. While the scholarship of discovery asks "what is known, what is yet to be found?" the scholarship of integrations asks "what do the findings *mean*?" (p. 19, italics original).

The last two types of scholarship proposed by Boyer may have been the most controversial. The "scholarship of application" suggests that, in order for research to be inherently useful, it must be applied in a useful way in service to a community. "How," asks Boyer, "can knowledge be applied to consequential problems?" (1990, p. 21). In many academic communities today, we would call this category of faculty work "service." Boyer places particular emphasis on the type of work that we as academics consider service because it typically is informed by our scholarship of discovery and integration. In other words, we use the knowledge that has been gained through disciplinary research to serve a local or national community.

The final category of scholarship that Boyer spent much of his energy expanding was the "scholarship of teaching" (1990, p. 23). He noted that "the work of the professor becomes consequential only as it is understood by others" (p. 23). In this view, teaching is an active process that expands the knowledge of the student and the teacher as well. The scholarship of teaching, Boyer argued, "means not only transmitting knowledge, but *transforming* and *extending* it" (p. 24). Teaching is a faculty responsibility that requires planning, reflection, and understanding. The scholarship of teaching is important, not only because it is good for the students' learning, but also because it attracts our future scholars and keeps the "flame of scholarship alive" (p. 24). In an age when faculty in our communication sciences and disorders (CSD) disciplines are at a premium, it may serve us well to focus our energies on SOTL, not only to improve our learners' outcomes, but to instill a love of learning in them such that they will go on to become faculty themselves. This may be the ultimate measure of our success as teachers.

In 1997, Lee S. Shulman succeeded Boyer as president of the Carnegie Foundation and continued advancing SOTL. Shulman suggested that, if the work of university teaching is to be valued, then it must be treated as "community property" (Shulman, 2004, p. 141). Just as real estate is valued, for example, because it is visible and comparable to other real-estate, teaching too must be visible. He noted (Shulman, 1998)

> A scholarship of teaching will entail a public account of some or all of the full act of teaching—vision, design, enactment, outcomes and analysis—in a manner susceptible to critical review by the teacher's professional peers and amenable to productive employment in future work by members of that same community. (p. 6)

In other words, we must make the act of teaching not only visible, but something to be judged by peers, just as the scholarship of discovery is peer reviewed in conference and publication contexts. For SOTL to serve the higher education community, we also must practice the scholarship of integration with the knowledge that we acquire regarding the teaching and learning process. That knowledge must be studied and applied by other faculty in higher education.

Dual Professions

Many faculty members in CSD programs might feel as though they have a split personality. That is, we serve as clinicians, researchers, and teachers. Many of us began our careers as clinicians and as such unhesitatingly filled in those occupation blanks on forms with "SLP." However, after joining the faculty at a university, we may find ourselves waffling as we fill in those occupation blanks. Are we "Speech Pathologists?" Or are we "Educators?" Our struggle with this issue may reflect the fact that in reality many of us are both.

Shulman (2004) calls on us to consider ourselves professional educators, no matter what our primary discipline may be. He notes that, in higher education, we take on the role and responsibility of educating those to whom we are passing on our disciplinary knowledge. As such, he advocates that engaging in SOTL is a critical mechanism for developing our teaching profession-selves. When we treat the work that we do in the classroom, the teaching and learning process, as "community property," we elevate the value of it by exposing it to peer review and by sharing it with others in our community to learn from and add on to (Shulman, 2004, p. 157). It is important to integrate this knowledge into our scholarly knowledge base by bringing the same level of critical inquiry to the teaching and learning that takes place in our classrooms as we bring to our disciplinary inquiries. In order for us to be truly effective as educators, we must endeavor to understand as much as we can about teaching and learning as we do about, say phonological processes or tympanography, and we must do so in a scholarly way.

The blending of our disciplinary knowledge and our knowledge of how to teach it is pedagogical content knowledge (PCK), and it represents the intersection of our two professions, as represented in Figure 1–1 (Shulman, 1987).

The concept of PCK was developed by Shulman in response to the recognition that, in the university setting, faculty often treat

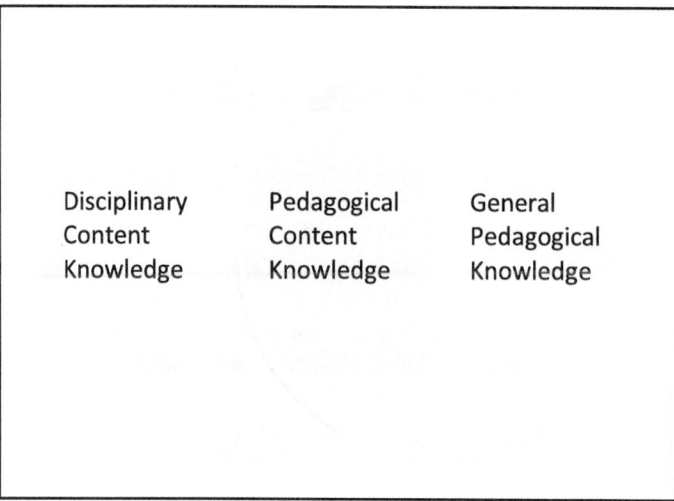

Figure 1–1. Pedagogical content knowledge.

our content knowledge and our knowledge about how to teach, or pedagogy, as mutually exclusive, separate entities. It represents the unique knowledge that content experts in our professions bring to the classroom when we skillfully craft learning experiences that are uniquely designed to make our content accessible for our learners, thereby transforming their knowledge. The PCK for different disciplines and professions is unique, as chemistry faculty will design learning experiences for chemistry students differently than audiology faculty will design learning for audiology students.

Our knowledge base as a professional speech-language pathologist (SLP) or audiologist is delineated clearly. We all come to our roles as clinicians and faculty with at least one graduate degree in the discipline. Additionally, in order to support our knowledge base and stay current with the research literature in our discipline, we engage in continuing education. We do this in part because the American Speech-Language-Hearing Association (ASHA) requires it of us and in part because we know how important it is to rely on the most recent evidence-based research available to guide our practice. As faculty in communication sciences and disorders (CSD), we are in the unique position of interacting with this evidence base in three ways:

1. We use this body of literature to guide us in teaching current knowledge to our students.
2. We rely on this material to guide any clinical practice we engage in, with or without our students.
3. We contribute to the body of evidence by conducting research and sharing it publically through peer-reviewed forums, such as conferences and publications.

By accepting Shulman's call on all faculty to be members of two professions—our own CSD profession and the profession of educator—we must consider what our educator knowledge base is, how we gather it, and how we maintain current knowledge. A few among us who have a knowledge base in education, or pedagogy, either because it was part of our disciplinary education, such as those of who were educated within a department of special education or who pursued teacher-certification as part of their studies. There are also a small, but lucky number of faculty who were formally prepared for teaching at a university during their doctoral program, such as those who participate in a "Preparing Future Faculty" program (Preparing Future Faculty, 2010). However, for the rest of us the path forward toward this knowledge is not always clear and simple. Despite the lack of formal training in this area, we still have a responsibility to provide the highest quality undergraduate and graduate education possible for our students. It is incumbent upon us to provide the most effective level of education for our students that we are capable of, but we need more information than we may have received in our doctoral programs about how to do this.

Because most of us did not come to our faculty positions adequately prepared to be professional educators, we must find alternative methods of gaining pedagogical knowledge and developing our own PCK for CSD. Although the wealth of information regarding effective higher education has been growing steadily over the past several decades, we are not always aware of it. Many faculty continue to rely on lectures as their principal approach to content delivery despite the evidence in the literature that lectures are not the most effective method of education. In fact, lectures, even when they are well designed, tend to be less effective for promoting problem solving, applying information to new situations, retaining content over extended periods of time, and improving affective learning outcomes than other active learning approaches (Fink, 2003). On their own, lectures may be adequate for transmitting information that will be retained for the short term, or until the end of the semester. Most of us likely would cite as learning goals for our students higher order learning outcomes, such as critical analysis and clinical problem solving. However, a good number of us are not all together clear about how to teach in a manner that will result in these outcomes.

We may perpetuate the overreliance on lecture for a variety of reasons. We may do so because of what Shulman refers to as the "impoverished model of apprenticeship" (Shulman, 2004, p. 230). We tend to teach as we were taught, as though, by being graduate students, we were apprentices to the teaching process. It is unlikely that we rely on lecturers out of apathy toward learning outcomes. In fact, we may be unaware of the ineffectiveness or shortcomings of lecturers. However, if we expect our students to become accomplished problem solvers and critical thinkers, particularly as clinicians, it only makes sense that we develop and utilize methods of teaching that we know will improve their abilities in this regard.

Doctoral programs tend to focus on teaching us the content in which we will become experts by the time we complete the degree. Universities hire us for that very content knowledge. And yet, we typically are asked during the interview process to provide an exemplar lecture as a point of evaluation. This is one of the few times we allow ourselves to be scrutinized as teachers. As we watch our potential, future colleague teach, what are we looking for? Likely, most of us are looking for factual accuracy. Did he describe the workings of the inner ear correctly? Does she know what the "p" in *p*-value means and indicates? How many of us are scrutinizing the interviewees' lectures for the quality of their delivery and their use of some method other than lecture? Although no data may be available to answer this, we could hazard a guess that based on anecdotal evidence the numbers are low. Many of us may not be familiar with what alternatives to lecture are most effective. We may not be in a position to judge others' effective teaching because we are not truly sure what effective teaching is.

Professional Educator Continuing Education

If we are to accept the responsibility for being a professional educator as well as a professional speech-language pathologist or audiologist, we must also accept responsibility for our own knowledge in the realm of education. "Why SOTL?" some may ask. The answer is because SOTL is what informs our knowledge about effective teaching, particularly in higher education. Through the use of and participation in SOTL, we grow our understanding of how to teach more effectively for particular types of content, how learners perceive our efforts, and how to create "significant learning" (Fink, 2003). It is our responsibility to teach as effectively as possible and understand what that means for our own classrooms. The question that may be looming, however, is just how do we do this?

One way for us to conceptualize our continuing education as professional educators is to consider how we might make use of SOTL work relative to where we are in our own development. ASHA creates mechanisms that make it easy for us to obtain continuing education in a variety of settings and topics. For just about any knowledge or skill listed within our scope of practice, we can attend free-standing workshops, seminars at conventions, read texts followed by quizzes, and participate in webinars online that allow us to keep our skills and knowledge current. However, if we are to consider our knowledge and skills in education under the same model, we would find little formal guidance or direction available as there is no governing body that is the equivalent of ASHA for our professional educator-selves.

Some faculty find themselves teaching on a campus that houses a center that will help improve teaching by learning about effective, new ways to teach beyond lectures. These centers often are called "centers for teaching excellence," "centers for teaching and learning," or "faculty development centers." Some faculty may bristle at the notion of consulting one of these centers, either because they do not believe that their skills need to be "developed" or because doing so may suggest that there is a problem with their teaching that needs to be fixed. Some stigma may be attached among some colleagues that seeking help for teaching implies bad teaching. On the other hand, identifying a problem in one's teaching may be an opportunity for reflection and exploration of the teaching and learning that is taking place in your class rather than being considered a professional flaw. Centers for teaching and learning can provide individual consultation to discuss perceived problems or concerns with teaching; they may offer structured workshops that provide small groups of faculty with information for effective teaching strategies; and they may sponsor seminars that are designed to support faculty as they move forward in developing their own agenda in SOTL research. No matter what modes of support a center offers, research and literature from SOTL likely will be at the heart of the content and can be used to support faculty at all levels of their development.

If no teaching and learning centers (TLC) are at an institution, it may be up to individuals to take on their professional educator continuing education. In this case, faculty members may need to work on their own or in small groups of colleagues to move their knowledge forward incrementally. Although the guidance of a faculty consultant, or developer, can ease this process, it is by no means an impossible undertaking without one. Here, we describe the different levels of educator skill development and possibilities of how to use SOTL work as you consider how to move through them and how far you want to proceed. Section II of this book includes a great deal of the information you need for the first stage of development as you reflect on your current teaching.

A Framework of Educator Development

Whereas ASHA CEU materials often are labeled "introductory," "intermediate," or "advanced level," we can consider a parallel framework for the level advancement in our teaching skills. One model that is useful for many faculty is McKinney's distinctions of *good teaching, scholarly teaching, and scholarship of teaching and learning* (McKinney, 2004). Although not strictly commensurate with the implications of ASHA's terms, these distinctions ring true for faculty at various stages of their development. We can describe where on the continuum of professional educator development each stage is in order for readers to begin identifying where they currently fit within this progression.

Good Teaching

McKinney (2007, p. 9) describes good teaching as "that which promotes student learning and other desired student outcomes." We believe that the vast majority of faculty start here. Most doctoral students participating in teaching experiences and new faculty begin with basic knowledge about what they received in the way of education when they were students. In the good teaching category, reflection is key. Reflections may focus on their own learning experience, as noted previously, or they may focus on what is happening in their current classrooms. Teachers at this point on the continuum attend to their feelings about a class and may think about what went well, what went poorly, and how to revise the parts that they aren't pleased with so as to improve the learning the next time. Simple reflection and observation can result in positive changes. The good teacher is one who cares about his or her teaching and works to make it as good as possible with a limited number of tools to make changes.

Scholarly Teaching

Those who take the same scholarly approach to teaching as they do to their clinical practice are considered in the stage of scholarly teaching. Reminiscent of Shulman's call for all of us in higher education to be professional educators, we bring a special type of scholarly thinking to teaching at this point. Faculty at this stage have some familiarity with the literature relevant to their approaches to teaching. Much as we are familiar with the literature that guides assessment of children for language delays or hearing loss, scholarly faculty are familiar with the literature regarding different types of assessments for learning, for example. McKinney notes that "scholarly teaching involves taking a scholarly approach to teaching just as we would take a scholarly approach to other areas of knowledge and practice" (McKinney, 2007, p. 9).

This does not mean that scholarly teachers are intimately familiar with all of the relevant research that produced the standard of best practice, but that they are reasonably knowledgeable about some best practice based on the literature. Many educators in speech-language pathology and audiology programs, for example, are familiar with the model of assessment that includes both formative and summative assessments without necessarily being familiar with the work of John Carroll from the 1970s that first described this approach to evaluation (Carroll, 1971). Knowledge at this stage builds from the literature such that teachers are developing familiarity with some of the SOTL research. What is important at this stage is the knowledge an applicable standard of practice informs us of what has been demonstrated in the literature to be effective.

Scholarship of Teaching and Learning

The farthest point on the continuum (McKinney, 2007) is the set of faculty who are engaging in SOTL. Teachers at this stage start to move beyond just reviewing the pertinent literature and begin to engage in a "process by which scholars prepare for their inquiry" and then begin the inquiry (Bernstein & Ginsberg, 2009, p. 45). At this stage, faculty often have combined their reflections from their time as good teachers with the knowledge base from their time as scholarly teachers to develop their own inquiries regarding teaching and learning. Often teachers who are beginning to consider engaging in SOTL have begun to recognize a teaching problem for which they have no answer.

In his ground-breaking article, Bass (1999) highlights that when we identify a problem within the context of our discipline, this often is considered a good thing as now the research can be designed and the scholarship of discovery can move forward. Regrettably, for many, identifying a problem in teaching is not a cause for excitement, but is perceived as something one should hide from colleagues, lest we are discovered to be an ineffective teacher. Consistent with Shulman, Bass argues that a problem in teaching presents the same opportunity as a research problem in that we can move forward with designing research that will increase our understanding of teaching and learning. Teachers in this stage are designing studies about teaching and learning, collecting data, and disseminating results publically about what they have learned. Recognition of this unique and valuable opportunity for participating in teaching and learning research, as well as the opportunity to contribute to the body of evidence regarding effective teaching, propel faculty to this stage.

Developing as Professional Educators: Working Toward Each Level

The purpose of professional educator development in higher education varies by individual goals and by framework/literature perspective. Some models, as noted previously, are relatively linear and consider that all development leads toward SOTL and describe the development of faculty knowledge as a straight continuum (Figure 1–2).

Another model (Bernstein & Ginsberg, 2009) views the continuum as a continuous cycle in which faculty at each stage play a valuable role in fueling the knowledge development of teachers in other

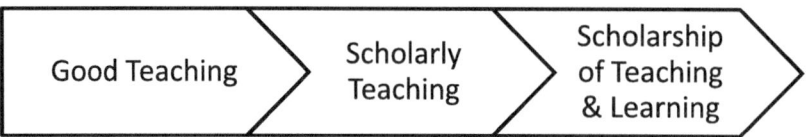

Figure 1–2. Linear progression toward SOTL.

stages of development. Whether subscribing to the linear or cyclical model of educator development, what may be most important to recognize is that not all teachers will necessarily have the desire to move to engaging in SOTL (Ginsberg, 2010).

We also can be at different junctures of development for different areas of knowledge. A teacher may have learned about authentic assessment through the literature and from conducting a study of assessment efficacy in her phonological disorders class, but have yet to begin to explore issues of technology in teaching. Although we are beginning to engage in SOTL for some aspects of teaching, we still may identify ourselves as being a scholarly teacher, yet to engage in SOTL, for other aspects of instruction. This model is consistent with Weston and McAlpine's (2001) notion that, although some activities are critical for forward movement of educator development, not all activities within a given phase must be completed for an individual to advance along the continuum. Weston and McAlpine describe a model, which like McKinney, treats SOTL as a possible end point in a continuum. Their phases of development are Phase 1: Growth in own teaching; Phase 2: Dialogue with colleagues about teaching and learning; and Phase 3: Growth in scholarship of teaching. They note, however, that teachers may develop in several ways, "within a phase, indicating a growth in complexity; and across phases, indicating a growth toward scholarship" (p. 90). In their model, they describe the teachers' evolving view of their role as educators and the steps that faculty may engage in to advance their knowledge and teaching.

Bernstein and Ginsberg (2009) suggest that the stages of development described by McKinney (2007) converge with Weston and McAlpine's continuum of growth (Weston & McAlpine, 2001) (see Figure 1–3). McKinney describes the destinations for professional

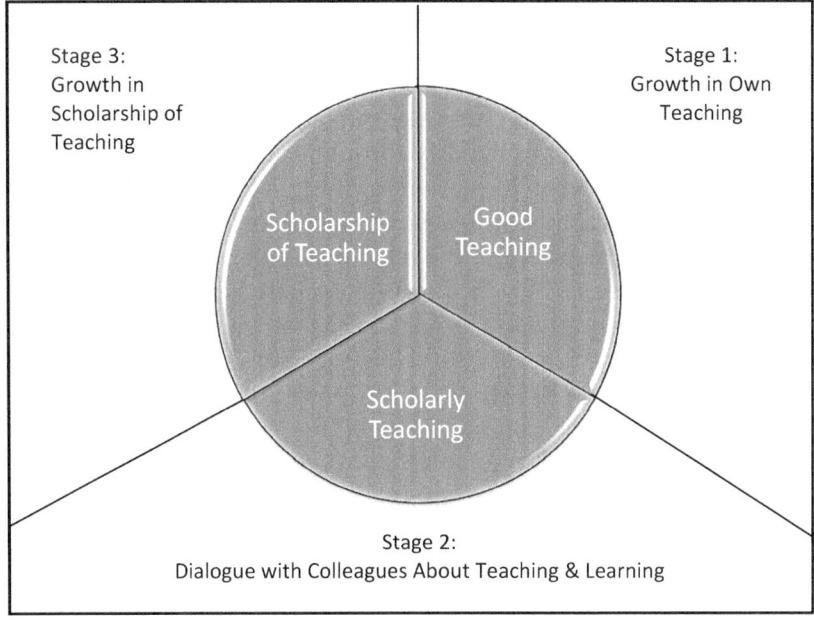

Figure 1-3. Integrated model of SOTL and faculty development. From "Toward an Integrated Model of the Scholarship of Teaching and Learning and Faculty Development" by Bernstein & Ginsberg, 2009, *Journal on Centers for Teaching & Learning*, *1*, p. 47. Copyright 2009 by Miami University. Reprinted with permission.

educator development as phases of *good teaching, scholarly teaching, and scholarship of teaching*. Weston and McAlpine focus on the behaviors and activities that characterize faculty in each stage of development, *growth in one's own teaching, dialogue about teaching and learning,* and *growth in scholarship of teaching and learning*. Bernstein and Ginsberg overlay the two models to highlight the relationship between the development destination and the activities associated with movement toward each destination. For our purposes, we will share some examples of activities that likely would advance the growth of professors at each phase of their development toward the stages of teaching skill. We use this framework to describe educator professional development in the following section.

Growing as Good Teachers

As noted previously, teachers in the early phases of their careers, including doctoral students, seldom are educated specifically regarding pedagogy, particularly for higher education. Teachers in this phase, called "growth in own teaching" (Weston & McAlpine, 2001, p. 91), are becoming increasingly aware of their teaching practices, students' learning, and the relationship between the two (Bernstein & Ginsberg, 2009). As a result, teachers who are growing in the category of good teachers are likely to engage in reflection on their teaching experiences, both while they are students and as new teachers, to develop (Weston & McAlpine, 2001). Although many of us, as noted previously, spent more than our fair share receiving knowledge through transmission-oriented lectures, we also had teachers who stand out in our minds as being particularly effective.

Most of us, with just a little reflection, will recall those positive learning experiences and try to emulate them to the best of our ability. As you recall one of your favorite teachers, think about what characteristic of theirs and their teaching stands out in your mind. It may be the teacher who let you discover some concept on your own, before telling you how to conceptualize of a new idea. It might have been the teacher who attempted to shape your powers of observation by asking to observe and report, giving you multiple opportunities to figure out how to do it rather than giving you a failing grade because you didn't do it right on the first try. Or it might be the teacher who delivered only lectures, but whose lectures were so straightforward, filled with examples and opportunities for dialogue, that you learned what a great lecture feels like. Faculty can be good teachers without being able to articulate specific learning theories that they subscribe to (Smith, 2001). Without knowledge of pedagogy, instructors can be very perceptive regarding students' reactions to teaching methods. For teachers who are attuned to basic student reactions, such as extreme quiet, negative body language, or looks of confusion, there is no need to be well-versed in theory to know that something needs to change in the delivery of the content. It may be a process of trial and error, something that we all go through, to find the right approach that results in boisterous discussions, positive body language, and enthusiasm for the topic in our class.

In addition to reflection, teachers in this phase may engage in other activities to support their teaching, whether independently or in the context of a TLC. For faculty who have access to a TLC, often a number of activities may be useful. If, as a faculty member, you decide to venture into a TLC, you likely will find they offer support with teaching evaluations. Although many schools utilize student evaluations of teaching as part of their tenure and promotion decision making, it sometimes is difficult for new teachers to interpret the results of student evaluations of teaching.

A TLC can be instrumental in helping faculty understand not only how to interpret their evaluations, but how to make changes that will improve students' evaluations. This is valuable, not only for improving teaching, but also for helping the tenure and promotion process. Sometimes we receive feedback that shows students think we are not "motivating" them sufficiently, but it may not be clear what we need to do in order to motivate them more. A TLC consultant can provide direction in how to improve this in the classroom because they are familiar with the SOTL literature. One of the values of a TLC consultant is that they can distill the knowledge that is available in the research that is directly applicable to the specific scenario that the teacher is dealing with such that the teacher does not have to begin the process of searching for the literature themselves in this phase of development.

In addition to providing interpretive assistance with end-of-semester course evaluations, TLC staff may offer mid-term course evaluations to provide the instructors with feedback that they can use right away, rather than after the term has ended and they are preparing for a new term. These mid-term evaluations, conducted by an outside person, can be immensely valuable to saving a course that seems to be heading in the wrong direction with no clear reason as to why. You can expect the TLC consultant to distribute questionnaires or feedback forms to the students in your absence and possibly conduct a focus group discussion to gather more specific feedback. They then will consolidate the information gathered, sit down with you, and talk about strengths, needs, and changes you might consider making, either currently or for the next time that you teach the class.

Mid-term assessments of the teacher and the course can help the teacher improve some small aspect of their teaching, such as identifying that a vocabulary list of new terms would be helpful to the students. Additionally, mid-term evaluations can be powerful opportunities for teachers and students alike to mutually share feedback. Many students may expect the end of the semester and recognize it as a compulsory process. Students are likely to understand the voluntary nature of the mid-term evaluation opportunity. This can be further enhanced by the instructor explicitly stating that the mid-course evaluation is being conducted in order for the instructor to make changes as needed right away to better improve students' learning. As the teacher receives feedback, he or she will reflect privately on the value and validity of student feedback. Decisions will be made to make small changes to some aspects of teaching or the class or to not change other aspects that were commented on by the students. As the teacher returns to the classroom following the capture of mid-semester feedback received from the TLC consultant, they have the opportunity to share with students that they not only appreciated their feedback, but what changes, if any, will happen as a result. Teachers also have the opportunity to explain to students what changes won't happen and why. This can become a very valuable dialogue that helps teachers and students alike come to a mutual understanding about what is happening in the class and why. For more information regarding the value of this type of communication, see Chapter 5.

If you find yourself teaching at an institution that does not have a TLC, you can still do plenty to make progress toward good teaching. Mid-term evaluations of the type the TLC can conduct, described previously, can be implemented easily without help in your classroom. One easy way to do this is to distribute blank index cards to your students and write three questions on the board for them to answer:

1. What happens in this class that supports my learning?
2. What happens in this class that hinders my learning?
3. What would I like to see more of in this class?

Tell them that these are anonymous, so they need not put their names on the cards unless they would like for you to follow up with them personally. As you collect the cards, let the students know that you will read all of their comments and will discuss with them the following week. Then after reading, considering, and deciding what you want to do with the feedback, bring it back to them as described previously. This process not only provides the opportunity for discussion about the teaching and learning process, it signals to your students that you care about their perceptions and their learning.

If you are not comfortable or aren't quite ready to undertake an independent mid-term evaluation in your class, but are looking for another mechanism for improving your teaching, consider observing a peer. This peer need not be in your program or in your department. Although Shulman suggests that each discipline has its own unique PCK that is rooted in the discipline and that SOTL also should be discipline specific (Shulman, 1987, 2004), Weimer argues that good teaching, and SOTL, shares more similarities across disciplinary boundaries than differences (Weimer, 2008). We would suggest that we have a great deal to learn by observing our colleagues teach. Unfortunately, with the busy and demanding schedules of academia, we often don't make time for visiting other teachers' classrooms and, indeed, some may even be resistant to it. We stand to learn about good teaching through observation, particularly while we are not in a student role. Sitting in the back of a good class and observing how the teacher engages the students in discussion, how she creates opportunities for active learning, or how he structures his teaching in a manner that is easy for students to follow is a wonderful use of an hour of your time. Figure 1–4 illustrates some basic steps for observing colleagues teaching. In Chapter 8 we examine a more formalized process of peer observations of teaching.

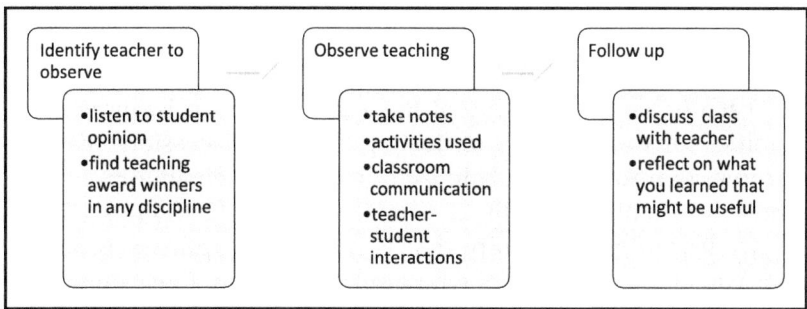

Figure 1–4. Observing Colleagues Teaching.

Growing as Scholarly Teachers

The second phase described by Weston and McAlpine (2001, p. 91) is labeled as "dialogue with colleagues about teaching and learning" and growth in this phase moves teachers toward scholarly teaching (Bernstein & Ginsberg, 2009; McKinney, 2004). The key difference in activities from the previous phase during which newer faculty consult more experienced colleagues and the sharing is relatively unidirectional. In this phase, the interactions between colleagues are more mutual, engaging in a sharing of ideas to "co-construct a more complex understanding of pedagogical content knowledge within their discipline and more generic knowledge of teaching across disciplines" (Weston & McAlpine, 2001, p. 92).

For faculty who have a TLC available to them, they may find that the faculty consultants staffing the center may be good colleagues to engage in these dialogues with. One of the advantages of engaging in such a dialogue with a faculty consultant is that this person often has broad knowledge of the SOTL literature that may be useful to you, and can make recommendations of materials to read to increase knowledge. By accessing the SOTL literature directly with guidance from a consultant, faculty in this phase begin to develop their own scholarly knowledge base of teaching in a relatively efficient manner. For example, if a faculty member is looking to identify mechanisms for integrating technology into teaching effectively, the TLC consultant can direct him to specific pieces of evidence-based education data from the SOTL literature without the teacher having to spend lengthy periods of time searching through all of the existing literature databases. This development of scholarly knowledge fosters in the teacher who is growing in this phase an ability to participate in dialogue, not just learn from those who are more experienced.

Faculty also may find that the TLC has set up learning communities for the purposes of hosting focused discussions. Faculty learning communities can help faculty develop their abilities toward scholarly teaching (Richlin & Cox, 2004). Cox (2001) describes a faculty learning community that is a cross-disciplinary group of approximately 11 members who are "engaged in a year-long program with curriculum about enhancing teaching and learning and with frequent seminars and activities that provide learning, development, and community building" (p. 71). Faculty learning communities are effective because, like students, teachers benefit from the opportunity to read, learn, discuss, and interact with each other (Cox, 2001).

Faculty learning communities based on Cox's model typically are focused in one of two ways. They can be cohort-focused. A cohort-focused group, as described by Cox (2001) originally was intended to identify a cohort of faculty who are in particular need of support due to isolation or other challenges. A common cohort that might benefit from such a learning community is new or junior faculty; rather than focusing on a single theme or teaching issue, the curriculum can encompass a number of broad issues that affect those new to academia, such as managing service time commitments and successfully applying for tenure. Alternatively, learning communities can be issue focused, in which case the curriculum addresses a specific topic, such as how to teach clinical problem solving or multicultural issues in education. A variety of members may be attracted to the specific theme from diverse backgrounds and all come together to address the issue as it pertains to their program or their role.

A key issue for faculty learning communities, across campus as well as in CSD, is likely to be scholarly teaching and SOTL literature. Although the prototype community described previously includes faculty from across a variety of disciplines, this is most feasible at a university where a TLC exists. If you are growing as a scholarly teacher without the support of a TLC, it may be possible to form your own community within your department to begin the exploration of SOTL material with the support and encouragement of colleagues. Your community may not follow the traditional model but may be adaptable for your purposes. In this case, you will need to choose a text that could serve for the foundation of your issue-focused curriculum. Several possibilities would include texts that cover a wide variety of evidence-based educational practices, such as collaborative learning strategies and designing effective writing assignments. Books we might suggest for this purpose would include Davis's *Tools for Teaching* (2009) and *McKeachie's Teaching Tips: Strategies, Research, and Theory for College and University Teachers* (Svinicki & McKeachie, 2010).

Key activities suggested by Cox (2001) then could be structured by a voluntary facilitator who would organize regular meetings in which the group gets together and discusses what they are reading and look for opportunities to expand knowledge beyond the boundaries of the group, such as finding related conferences to attend. Additionally, members of the group might consider taking on projects or activities that reflect their interest in scholarly teaching and extend their knowledge by incorporating the projects in their own classrooms. Participating in a learning community, whether formally organized by a TLC unit or undertaken by a group of like-minded colleagues, will support development in the growth of scholarly teaching.

Growing in Scholarship of Teaching and Learning

The final phase of development described by Weston and McAlpine (2001) is Phase 3: Growth in scholarship of teaching during which time faculty are moving toward engaging in SOTL. Again, we think it is important to emphasize that we are not suggesting that all faculty will want to or should conduct SOTL investigations. For faculty whose research agendas are so full with disciplinary specific research, or for faculty who are still working toward tenure and SOTL research will not be rewarded in the process by their institution, then participating in SOTL research may not be feasible. No judgment should be implied or inflicted on those who choose not to pursue SOTL as part of their own scholarly agendas. For faculty who choose to develop SOTL, it may be that the naturally inquisitive nature that propels us to undertake doctoral studies and research in our fields will drive us to apply the same inquiry process to increase our understanding of teaching and learning, which is what this phase is really all about (Weston & McAlpine, 2001). Further, faculty increasing their development in SOTL will be propelled by the same scholarly instincts that have gotten them this far to disseminate their work and subject it to peer-review, as Shulman advocates.

Opportunities for activities that support faculty beginning to participate in SOTL work may or may not be structured through TLC programs. Where TLCs operate, they can support faculty in this phase by providing them with resources, such as release-time or honorariums to participate in year-long seminars (Bernstein &

Ginsberg, 2009; Richlin & Cox, 2004). The seminar can provide not only time or funding to support SOTL endeavors, but it also can provide structured facilitation by an experienced SOTL researcher that will help them be successful as they undertake this new line of research for the first time.

Additionally, the TLC can offer faculty learning communities of the type described previously with an issue-focused theme of engaging in SOTL. In this case, teacher projects that individual participants may undertake would include the design and implementation of SOTL studies, with the expectation of public dissemination at the end of the time frame (Cox, 2001). Campus TLCs also can bring SOTL speakers to campus, from nearby colleges and universities or by funding a well-known speaker. Bringing a speaker to a campus can be a cost-effective way of sharing information with a large number of interested faculty, as well as inciting and instilling more curiosity in those who have yet to begin their journey from the early stage of good teaching (Bernstein & Ginsberg, 2009).

As with the previous two phases, many opportunities are available to grow in SOTL without the support of a TLC. Faculty can form their own learning community, with members of the CSD faculty or with faculty from across campus, that focus the issue of SOTL. If this option is being considered, texts that would serve well as the foundation for the curriculum might include *Teaching as Community Property* (Shulman, 2004) or *Enhancing Learning Through the Scholarship of Teaching and Learning* (McKinney, 2007). Unlike the Davis and McKeachie texts, these texts will move the readers' thinking further forward to developing their own line of inquiry within SOTL. Weekly or biweekly meetings to discuss these thought-provoking texts, in addition to other readings, will be valuable to enhancing understanding and application of the material. Individual members will want to develop their own SOTL investigations, much as they would if they were participating in a TLC supported learning community. Additionally, attendance at related SOTL conferences likely will be requisite and very valuable, not only for the opportunity to extend the community, form networks, and learn from colleagues, but also for the purpose of making public results and knowledge gained (Bernstein & Ginsberg, 2009; Richlin & Cox, 2004; Weston & McAlpine, 2001).

Finally, a note regarding the growth cycle for those who are moving beyond their good teaching stage and are becoming scholarly teachers or teachers engaged in SOTL. Several models of professional development in higher education described here (Bernstein & Ginsberg, 2009; Cox, 2001; Weston & McAlpine, 2001) suggest that faculty who have advanced their SOTL knowledge have a responsibility and a role in mentoring those who have yet to get there. The faculty learning community model describes the value of senior faculty mentoring more junior faculty (Cox, 2001). Bernstein and Ginsberg suggest that the way to support growth of faculty in effective teaching on a campus is to provide opportunities for faculty developing at different stages to interact in such a way as to stimulate discussion and learning for everyone. Weston and McAlpine (2001) describe the teachers undertaking growth in the scholarship of teaching as taking on mentoring roles, becoming leaders on their campus. Whichever model appeals to you, we must adopt the position that teaching is part of our professional identity and that it is incumbent on us to be as effective as we can as educators. We would not, as professional speech-language pathologists and audiologists, accept the notion that we would provide clinical care to our clients that is less than effective or that we are less than capable of providing. As we make our way toward being professional educators, SOTL will play an invaluable role in getting us there.

References

Bass, R. (1999). The scholarship of teaching: What's the problem? *Inventio: Creative Thinking About Learning and Teaching, 1*(1), 1–10.

Bernstein, J., & Ginsberg, S. (2009). Toward an integrated model of the scholarship of teaching and learning and faculty development. *Journal of Centers for Teaching and Learning, 1*, 41–55.

Boyer, E. L. (1990). *Scholarship reconsidered: Priorities of the professoriate.* San Francisco, CA: Jossey-Bass.

Carroll, J. B. (1971). Problems of measurement related to the concept of learning for mastery. In J. Block (Ed.), *Mastery learning: Theory and practice* (pp. 29–45). New York, NY: Holt, Rinehart and Winston.

Cox, M. D. (2001). Faculty learning communities: Change agents for transforming institutions into learning organizations. In D. Lieberman & C. Wehlburg (Eds.), *To improve the academy No. 19*, (pp. 69–93). San Francisco, CA: Jossey-Bass.

Davis, B. G. (2009). *Tools for teaching*. San Francisco, CA: Jossey-Bass.

Fink, L. D. (2003). *Creating significant learning experiences*. San Francisco, CA: Jossey-Bass.

Ginsberg, S. M. (2010, August 31). Getting to the scholarship of teaching and learning: Professional development in university faculty. *The ASHA Leader,* pp. 14–17.

McKinney, K. (2004). The scholarship of teaching and learning: Past lessons, current challenges, and future visions. In C. M. Wehlburg & S. Chadwick-Blossey (Eds.), *To improve the academy: No. 22* (pp. 3–19). Bolton, MA: Anker.

McKinney, K. (2007). *Enhancing learning through the scholarship of teaching and learning*. Bolton, MA: Anker.

Preparing Future Faculty. (2010). *The Preparing Future Faculty program*. Retrieved from http://www.preparing-faculty.org/

Richlin, L., & Cox, M. (2004, Spring). Developing scholarly teaching and the scholarship of teaching and learning through faculty learning communities. In M. D. Cox & L. Richlin (Eds.), *New directions for teaching and learning, No. 97* (pp. 127–136). San Francisco, CA: Jossey-Bass.

Shulman, L. S. (2004). *Teaching as community property*. San Francisco, CA: Jossey-Bass.

Shulman, L. S. (1998). Introduction. In Pat Hutchings (Ed.), *The course portfolio: How faculty can examine their reaching to advance practice and improve student learning* (pp. 5–12). Sterling, VA: Stylus.

Shulman, L. S. (1987). Knowledge and teaching: Foundations of the new reform. *Harvard Educational Review, 36,* 1-22.

Smith, R. A. (2001). Expertise and the scholarship of teaching. In C. Kreber (Ed.), *New directions for teaching and learning: No. 86., Scholarship revisited: Perspectives on the scholarship of teaching and learning* (pp. 69–78). San Francisco, CA: Jossey-Bass.

Svinicki, M., & McKeachie, W. J. (2010). *McKeachie's teaching tips: Strategies, research, and theory for college and university teachers*. Belmont, CA: Wadsworth.

Weimer, M. (2008). Positioning scholarly work on teaching and learning. *International Journal for the Scholarship of Teaching and Learning, 2*(1). 1–6. Retrieved from http://www.georgiasouthern.edu/isotl

Weston, C. B., & McAlpine, L. (2001, Summer). Making explicit the development toward the scholarship of teaching. In C. Kreber (Ed.), *New directions for teaching and learning: No. 86. Scholarship revisited: Perspectives on the scholarship of teaching and learning* (pp. 89–98). San Francisco, CA: Jossey-Bass.

EBP in Clinical Practice versus EBE in Classroom Teaching

> *If a child can't learn the way we teach, maybe we should teach the way they learn.*
>
> —Ignacio Estrada

Evidence-Based Practice as the Foundation for Clinical Service Delivery

In our clinical lives as speech-language pathologists and audiologists, we strive to provide the best clinical services to our clients. To provide the best clinical services, we have been required to determine what is best based on the available clinical evidence. In 2005, the American Speech-Language-Hearing Association (ASHA) released a position statement on Evidence-Based Practice (EBP) in Communication Disorders. ASHA defined EBP as "an approach in which current, high-quality research evidence is integrated with practitioner expertise and client preferences and values into the process of making clinical decisions" (ASHA, 2005, p. 1). Dollaghan (2007) took the concepts of EBP and adapted them into what she terms E^3BP or the three types of evidence that are needed for EBP in Communication Sciences and Disorders (CSD). The three types of evidence are "(1) best available *external* evidence from systematic research, (2) best available evidence *internal* to clinical practice, and (3) best available evidence concerning the preferences of a fully informed patient" (Dollaghan, 2007, p. 2) (Figure 2–1). Therefore, clinicians must not only examine the external evidence from the published research, but they also must examine the internal evidence from their clinical experience with a specific client to determine the best approach to be utilized with that client. Furthermore, the clinician also needs to educate or inform the client in order to incorporate the client's informed preferences into the clinical decision-making process. Dollaghan goes on to explain that the E^{3}BP model does not specifically refer to "clinical expertise" because it is not a separate component to the model, "but rather the glue by which the best available evidence of all three kinds is integrated in providing optimal clinical care" (p. 3).

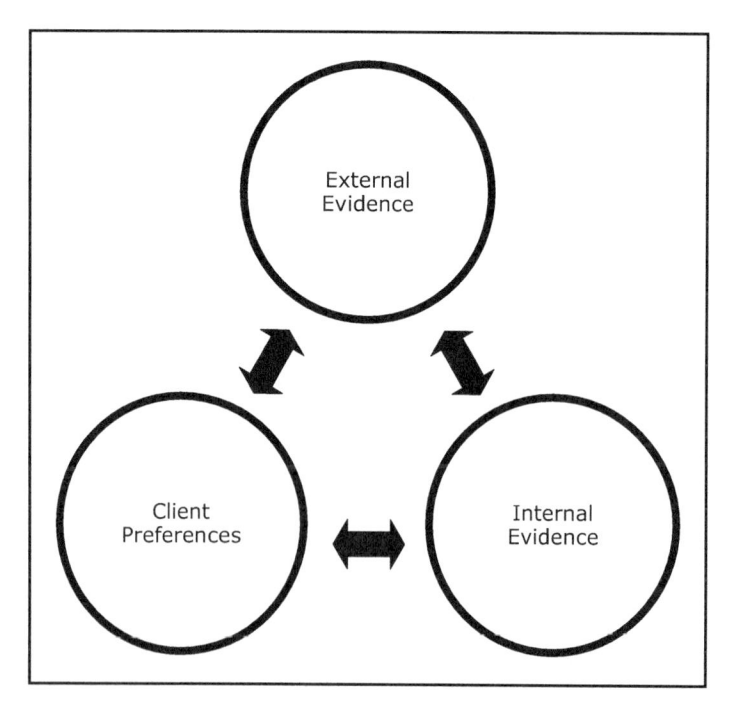

Figure 2–1. Elements of E^{3}BP. Based on Dollaghan (2007).

EBP Levels of Evidence

To determine the best available external evidence from the systematic clinical research, we need to examine the strength or levels of evidence. Many hierarchies exist for examining levels of evidence; therefore, for our purposes, we will use Robey's (2004) levels of evidence.

Level 1 evidence is the most rigorous and, thus, is more effective in its clinical use versus Level 4 evidence, which is less rigorous. Level 1 evidence is research based on randomized control trials (RCT). This is considered the strongest level of evidence available because the design is least susceptible to bias. In Level 1 studies, participants are randomly assigned to two or more different treatment groups (e.g., treatment group versus a control or no treatment group), and the study is strictly controlled for bias. The outcomes from each group are compared, and the results reported. Although RCT are considered the "gold standard" or the strongest evidence available, they may not be the most appropriate type of research for the question(s) being posed, ethical reasons, or the intervention approach being studied, among other reasons.

The next level of evidence may be more appropriate in some cases. Level 2 studies are well-designed studies; however, they are not randomized, but the researchers still control for bias. Level 2 studies include quasi-experimental studies in which the participants are not randomized to the conditions or groups, but the experimental procedures are still employed in the study. Therefore, the researcher does not have control of an independent variable because the intervention is already in process, or it was impossible or unethical to manipulate the variable (e.g., withholding treatment for the sake of the study). Thus, when comparisons are made, they are made on nonequivalent groups that may differ on more than just the treatment approach being examined.

A third level of evidence, Level 3, utilizes well-designed non-experimental studies such as correlational studies, case-control studies, observational research, survey research, and archival research. These studies lack the randomized conditions and the strict experimental procedures; however, they are useful in providing evidence when experimental research cannot be conducted for whatever reason.

The weakest level of evidence on the hierarchy is Level 4, which consists of expert committee reports, consensus conference, clinical experience of respected authorities, and observational studies. Some areas of research are limited to Level 4 evidence, but this is slowly changing as clinicians and researchers are actively working to improve the EBP research that is available.

With ASHA's 2005 position statement on EBP, professionals in the fields of CSD have actively worked to gather the evidence needed and to design research to establish the needed evidence from which to base our clinical practice. At this point in time, very limited Level 1 evidence exists, but we have improved beyond making clinical decisions based only on clinical experience of respected authorities (Level 4 evidence). In addition to improving the evidence that is available, the professions also have improved the accessibility of the evidence, as seen in the following resources:

- ASHA's *Compendium of EBP Guidelines and Systematic Reviews* (http://www.asha.org/members/ebp/compendium/)
- *Evidence-Based Practice Briefs* (http://www.speechandlanguage.com/ebp-briefs)
- LinguiSystems *Guide to Evidence-Based Practice* (http://www.linguisystems.com/pdf/EBPguide.pdf)
- National Center for Evidence-Based Practice (NCEP) (http://www.ncepmaps.org/)

The intentional pursuit of EBP research and accessibility to this research leads professionals to actively question what they are doing in the clinical setting and why they are doing it. This internal questioning leads to a more informed professional, which, in turn, should lead to better clinical outcomes for our clients.

Evidence-Based Education as the Foundation for Classroom Teaching

Similar to EBP within the clinical setting, we believe there is a need for faculty members to utilize Evidence-Based Education (EBE) within the educational setting. What is EBE? We propose that EBE is an educational approach in which current, high-quality scholarship of teaching and learning (SOTL) research evidence is integrated with pedagogical content knowledge (PCK) (Shulman, 1998) and teacher-learner interaction in making educational decisions in order to maximize student learning outcomes (Figure 2–2). Therefore, similar to the clinician basing their clinical decisions on E^3BP, the professor/instructor relies on the integration of the best available evidence from three key elements. The first element is the best available external evidence from systematic SOTL research within and across disciplines. SOTL provides the research evidence for the decisions we make as we plan and implement our classroom teaching. The next element is the best available evidence from internal evidence or PCK. As Shulman (1998) stated, PCK incorporates our content knowledge, which for us is our knowledge of the field of CSD, together with our knowledge about how to teach and how to teach that content. The third and final element of EBE is the best available evidence from the teacher-learner interaction. The teacher-learner interaction is a reciprocal process. From the professor's/instructor's viewpoint the

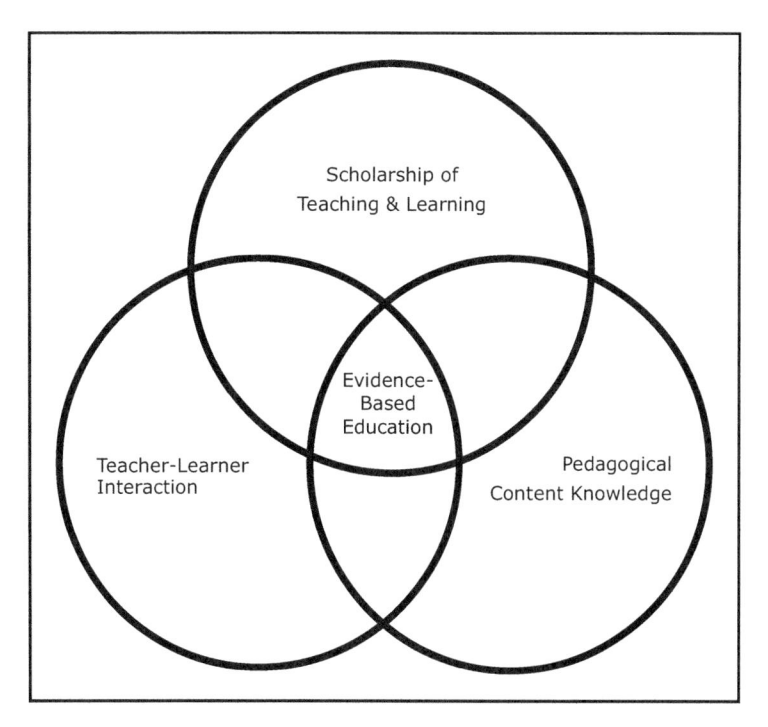

Figure 2–2. Elements of evidence-based education (EBE).

teacher-learner interaction includes information about the following demographic components of the students and the course, as well as factors related to individuals student perspectives:

- level that the students are at in their education (e.g., freshman, sophomores, juniors, seniors, master level graduate students, doctoral level students)
- student's background knowledge on the topic (e.g., limited or no background or foundational knowledge, some coursework in CSD, coursework and clinical experiences with CSD)
- types of students in the classroom (e.g., undergraduate non-majors, undergraduate majors, graduate students)
- type of college/university setting where the course is taught
- format of the course (e.g., online, reduced contact, traditional semester course, lab, etc.)
- students' reason for enrollment in the course (e.g., elective course, requirement for general education requirements, requirement for the major or minor)
- students' familiarity with professor/instructor (e.g., first class with professor/instructor, multiple classes with professor/instructor)
- student's perception of professor/instructor approachability, immediacy, or social presence
- students' motivational level to be successful in the course.

EBE, therefore, requires the professor/instructor to critically evaluate the best available evidence from SOTL, PCK, and teacher-learner interaction to provide the best educational experiences to the student(s) and maximize student learning outcomes. Although the relationship between these three elements could be represented similar to the triangular relationship of EBP, we feel that a more accurate representation is as three overlapping elements. This relationship reflects the overlapping relationship of the three elements to each other, and the importance of all three elements working together in order for EBE to be fully realized.

EBE Levels of Evidence

EBP presents a hierarchy for the various levels of evidence in which the clinician seeks out the highest level of evidence from which to base clinical decisions. In Weimer's (2006) book *Enhancing Scholarly Work on Teaching & Learning: Professional Literature That Makes a Difference*, she discusses approaches to classifying scholarly work on teaching. Weimer's analysis provides us with a hierarchy or levels of evidence from which we can examine the SOTL research. On one end of the continuum is what Weimer terms research scholarship, and at the other end is the wisdom-of-practice.

Research Scholarship

On one end of the continuum are three types of research scholarship: quantitative investigations, qualitative studies, and descriptive research (Weimer, 2006). Quantitative investigations utilize research methodology from the social sciences and educational research, whereby the research involves the manipulation of variables across or between a treatment group and a control group. The advantage of quantitative studies is the ability to draw casual conclusions (McKinney, 2007). Comparative studies are an example of a quantitative investigation, which involves an examination of the differences between groups (e.g., the effectiveness of a PowerPoint and lecture based approach versus an active learning approach to teaching on mastery of learning outcomes). Correlational studies examine the relationships between two or more variables. Although comparative and correlational studies can be quantitative investigations, more frequently they tend to be descriptive forms of research, which are discussed later in this section. In general, quantitative investigations utilize an experimental design that manipulates variables to answer or study a research question. The quantitative research approach has become more common in pedagogical research.

According to Weimer (2006), qualitative studies comprise the newest and smallest category of published work of the three types of research scholarship. However, its use and acceptance has grown in recent years. Qualitative research utilizes methodology from the disciplines of the social sciences and the humanities. Therefore, qualitative research systemically examines and interprets naturally occurring teaching and learning events. It tends to reflect the participant's perspective of the learning activity (McKinney, 2007). Some examples of qualitative research designs are conversational analysis examining student learning in a course, teacher experiences in the classroom, analysis of teacher-learner interactions during clinical experiences, or student perspectives regarding the use of a specific pedagogical approach, such as clickers, problem-based learning, or other active learning approaches. The research can occur as a case study, interview, or focus group of participants, course portfolios, or an analysis of course artifacts. The methods of analysis for qualitative research are frequently labor intensive, which may contribute to the limited amount of qualitative research available.

Descriptive research is the third and most popular methodological approach to research scholarship described by Weimer (2006). Descriptive research has been used to describe faculty beliefs and opinions about teaching and learning, student's attitudes regarding pedagogical approaches, the prevalence of pedagogical approaches, comparisons of faculty and student responses to course goals or learning outcomes, comparison of content of course textbooks, and so forth. The methodological approach used most frequently in descriptive research is the survey, which then allows for statistical analysis of the results.

Wisdom-of-Practice

The lowest level of evidence is the wisdom-of-practice, which is experience-based pedagogical scholarship that includes personal accounts of change, recommended-practices reports, recommended-content reports, and personal narratives. Personal account of change is scholarship that includes reports by faculty regarding their experience with implementing a change in "instructional policy, practice, technique, method, or approach" (Weimer, 2006, p.40). As Weimer goes on to explain, personal accounts may include a single technique implemented in a course (i.e., student-generated exam questions), a collection of teaching strategies (i.e., cooperative learning), or a course that utilized an entirely new approach or new philosophy on teaching or education (i.e., developing a new course with a new approach, new curriculum, or critical pedagogy). Therefore, personal accounts focus on *"what* is changed—not *why"* (p. 58).

Recommended-practice reports are advice about what should be done in specific aspects of instruction. Much of the advice is telling faculty what to do, whereas some are recommendations or suggestions as to how to teach. These reports can be based on a single faculty member in a specific course or can be based on the experiences of a group of faculty members either within or across disciplines. As Weimer (2006) points out, one of the most impressive recommended-practice reports is Boyer's (1990) discussion of the scholarships of integration and application. The scholarship of integration occurs when scholars interpret and make clear and/or intentional connections between the concepts and/or across disciplines that leads to new insights on the research (Boyer, 1990). On the other hand, the scholarship of application is a dynamic process in which a new understanding of the concepts occurs as a result of active engagement with or "application" of the information. The type of reports that are generated through the scholarship of integration and application are typically in the form of recommended-practice reports.

A third type of scholarship in the wisdom-of-practice is recommended-content reports. Similar to recommended-practice reports, recommended-content reports provide advice about teaching, not about the manner or practice of teaching, but rather about the content or specifically proposing ways "to explain, illustrate, demonstrate, and otherwise support the acquisition of course content" (Weimer, 2006, p. 41). In addition, these reports provide recommendations regarding the knowledge, skills, or professional perspectives that should be included within a curriculum for a specific program of study (i.e., ASHA's Knowledge and Skills Acquisition). This level of evidence overlaps with Shulman's (1987) concept of PCK.

Personal narratives are the fourth and final type of evidence in the wisdom-of-practice scholarship. More diversity exists in this area of research, in that the author tends to examine his own personal ideas of pedagogy or responses to other's views based on his personal viewpoint. Therefore, the scholarship in this area tends to be more emotionally based. As Weimer (2006) explains, examples of personal narratives include

> accounts of personal growth that track development or the evolution of pedagogical thought, individual statements of teaching philosophy, and work that expresses a particular point of view (faculty should not have to teach college students basic skills), argues for one side of an issue (students are not customers), takes a position (grading on a curve is wrong), or advocates for a change in more broadly based policy issues (more outcomes assessment would improve academic quality). (p. 42)

Therefore, within EBE, the levels of evidence range from the research scholarship to wisdom-of-practice. Each level is important and provides us with valuable information from which to base our educational decisions. Whether our educational decisions are based on quantitative experiments, qualitative studies, descriptive research, personal accounts, recommended-practice reports, recommended-content reports, or personal narratives, all of this evidence is important and should be utilized especially if our goal in teaching is to maximize student learning outcomes.

Linking the Levels of Evidence in EBP to EBE

Borrowing from the levels of evidence used in EBP, we propose that EBE also has a hierarchy of levels of evidence (Table 2–1). The strongest evidence in EBE would be Level 1 evidence, which consists of RCT. Level 1 studies would have participants/students who are randomly assigned to two or more different pedagogical groups (e.g., treatment group or "new pedagogical approach" versus a control group or "traditional classroom pedagogical approach"; problem-based learning versus lecture/discussion) and the study would be strictly controlled for bias. The learning outcomes from each group would be compared and the results reported. True experimental designs often are unrealistic due to the practical and ethical considerations (McKinney, 2007). Level 2 EBE evidence would consist of well-designed studies; however, they would not be randomized, and yet the researchers would still control for bias. Level 2 studies would include quantitative investigations in which the participants/students were not randomized to the pedagogical conditions or groups, but experimental procedures still would be employed in the study. Therefore, the researcher would not have control of an independent variable because the pedagogical approach was already in process, or it was impossible or unethical to manipulate the variable (e.g., withholding educational support for the sake of the study). The next level for EBE would be Level 3, which utilizes well-designed non-experimental studies, such as correlational studies, case studies, observational research, survey research, and archival research.

Table 2-1. Comparison of the Levels of Evidence for EBP and EBE

Level of Evidence	Evidence-Based Practice (EBP)	Evidence-Based Education (EBE)
1	High-quality randomized control trials (RCT)	
2	Control study without randomization; quasi-experimental studies	Quantitative investigations
3	Non-experimental studies; case-control studies; correlational studies; observational research with controls; survey research; and archival research	Qualitative studies Descriptive studies
4	Expert opinion; committee reports; consensus reports; clinical experience of respected authorities; observational studies without control	Wisdom-of-practice—personal accounts of change, recommended practice reports, recommended-content reports, personal narratives

These studies lack the randomized conditions and the strict experimental procedures; however, they are useful in providing evidence when experimental SOTL research cannot be conducted for whatever reason. Level 3 studies most likely would be qualitative studies and frequently are the starting point for many more well-controlled SOTL studies. Similar to EBP levels, the weakest level of evidence for EBE is Level 4 or studies in the category of the wisdom-of-practice. Therefore, the evidence would include personal accounts of change, recommended-practice reports, recommended-content reports, and personal narratives. Initial SOTL research frequently focused on Level 3 or 4 evidence, but this is beginning to change as educators embrace SOTL to improve their teaching and the learning outcomes.

Why Do We Need EBE?

We know that it is important to approach our clinical practices using EBP, but does it really matter whether we use EBE in our classroom? We believe that it does matter. If our goal as educators is to maximize learning in our students, then we need to use EBE to do so. If so, why are not more of us engaged in EBE and SOTL research? For most of us, the answer to that question may be that we do not have the time. Our professional lives require us to balance a full teaching load, content-specific research responsibilities, service commitments to the college/university and possibly beyond, and student advising. We cannot imagine adding anything else to the to-do list. For others, educational research or SOTL is not required and/or valued for promotion and tenure (see Chapter 9 for further discussion on this issue), so it just does not happen. Or maybe we assume that, because our professional training is in CSD, we are not prepared to do research on teaching. After all, we did not pursue higher education in pedagogy, rather our doctoral training is within a specialized area of speech-language pathology, audiology, speech science, or hearing science. Finally, we may believe that research will not help us in the classroom, or worse yet, that it may contradict the traditional educational approaches that we have been using throughout our careers.

Even if we do not have the opportunity to conduct SOTL research to contribute to EBE, we have a duty to use it to guide our educational practices. We believe that EBE is crucial for every educator to change and begin to consciously evaluate what is happening within his or her classroom; make conscious decisions about how to meet the learning outcomes for their students; and maximize student learning and retention of information. After all, for those of us already actively engaged in the use of EBP in our clinical lives, the use of EBE is not that different. We have the foundational knowledge and skills for utilizing evidence. We just need to move it from the clinical environment to the classroom environment.

When incorporating EBP into our clinical lives, we start by formulating our EBP question that is based on our client and the presenting communication deficit(s). From there, we utilize our clinical knowledge of the client's presenting deficits and knowledge of communication disorders. We then search for research that provides us with treatment evidence for the communication deficit. After we have gathered the evidence, we critically evaluate the evidence, utilizing our clinical knowledge and knowledge of the client. We also gather information from the client regarding their preferences, values, and needs. Based on the three elements of evidence, external research, internal clinical knowledge, and the informed client, we determine the intervention approach to be utilized. As we incorporate that intervention approach into our practice, we monitor the client's progress and make changes as needed in order to provide the best clinical services for that client.

We can take the same approach as we move to incorporate EBE into our academic lives. We begin by examining the course to be taught and the students in the course. Specifically, we utilize our PCK and begin asking ourselves many questions. What is the content being taught? What are the learning outcomes? How can I teach the content? What are my options for teaching the content? What, if any, technology should I use? What examples, demonstrations, analogies, comparisons, illustrations, or activities might be useful in teaching that content? From there, we examine the teacher-learner interaction by asking questions from both the teacher perspective and our view of the student's perspective. Therefore, we would ask questions such as: Who are the students? What is their background knowledge for the course? Are they undergraduate students, graduate students, majors in communication disorders, or majors in some other discipline? Why might the student be enrolled in the course? What is the student's motivation for taking the course? How do I need to approach the content given the student's perspective and motivation?

The final element to consider in applying EBE to the classroom is to examine the SOTL research. We need to determine what the research says about teaching and learning and how to maximize student learning outcomes. Based on the three elements of evidence for education—PCK, teacher-learner interaction, and SOTL research—we determine the pedagogical approach(es) to utilize for that specific course. As we incorporate that pedagogical approach(es) into our classroom, we monitor the student's progress on learning outcomes and make appropriate changes as needed to provide students with the best educational experience and to maximize student learning outcomes.

Where Do I Find the Evidence?

By now, we hope you understand the importance of approaching teaching based on EBE. You are ready to examine your course. The easy part is to start with your PCK and teacher-learner interaction. These are elements that you can address without much external information. The more difficult part is to examine the SOTL research. If you have not done that before, you may be asking "Where do I find SOTL research?" SOTL research has been expanding over the years. Because it would be impossible to provide an exhaustive list of SOTL resources, we have provided a few SOTL resources that we have found to be a good starting point for SOTL.

- Carnegie Foundation for the Advancement of Teaching (www.carnegiefoundation.org)
- *International Journal for the Scholarship of Teaching and Learning* (www.georgiasouthern.edu/ijsotl)
- International Society for the Scholarship of Teaching and Learning (www.issotl.org)
- *Journal of the Scholarship of Teaching and Learning* (www.iupui.edu/~josotl)
- The Carnegie Academy for the Scholarship of Teaching and Learning (CASTL) in Higher Education (http://gallery.carnegie foundation.org/gallery_of_tl/castl_he.html)
- *The Teaching Professor* (www.teachingprofessor.com)

Now What Do I Do?

So EBE sounds like a good idea, but how do you go about incorporating it into your classroom? The next chapter introduces you to some foundational teaching concepts that are evidence-based in nature. This chapter lays the foundation for the remainder of the book as we move you through EBE practices, the mechanisms for engaging in SOTL, course design, assessment, and designing SOTL research.

References

American Speech-Language-Hearing Association. (2005). *Evidence-based practice in communication disorders* [Position Statement]. Available from www.asha.org/policy

Boyer, E. L. (1990). *Scholarship reconsidered: Priorities of the professoriate.* San Francisco, CA: Jossey-Bass.

Dollaghan, C. A. (2007). *Communication evidence-based practice in communication disorders.* Baltimore, MD: Paul H. Brookes.

McKinney, K. (2007). *Enhancing learning through the scholarship of teaching and learning: The challenges and joys of juggling.* San Francisco, CA: Anker.

Robey, R. R. (2004, April 13). Levels of evidence. *The ASHA Leader.* Retrieved from http://www.asha.org/Publications/leader/2004/040413/f040412a2.htm

Shulman, L. S. (1987). Knowledge and teaching: Foundations of the new reform. *Harvard Educational Review, 57*(1), 1–22.

Shulman, L. S. (1998). Introduction. In Pat Hutchings (Ed.), *The course portfolio: How faculty can examine their teaching to advance practice and improve student learning* (pp. 5–12). Sterling, VA: Stylus.

Weimer, M. (2006). *Enhancing scholarly work on teaching and learning: Professional literature that makes a difference.* San Francisco, CA: Jossey-Bass.

The "Learner Centered-Active Learning" Paradigm

> *Tell me and I'll forget; show me and I may remember; involve me and I'll understand.*
>
> —Chinese Proverb

Undoubtedly, many faculty have memories of their "best" or "most effective" teachers. We recall these individuals fondly because they made an impact on us as learners for one reason or another. Why is that? How did they help to engage us and facilitate our understanding of a particular topic in such a memorable way? Perhaps their general style of classroom management was stellar, or our favorite teachers were able to actively involve students in the learning process. Whatever the case, many would argue that new faculty attempt to emulate the most successful characteristics of their favored course instructors as they begin their own teaching careers. This is not a bad practice, *per se*; however it is critical to ensure that the teaching behaviors we strive to emulate are grounded in evidence-based education (EBE) practices. This is complicated by the fact that many new faculty begin their teaching careers having little instruction on *how* to teach or what constitutes EBE. We are all subject matter specialists who research and/or practice clinically in our discipline-specific areas of interest, but lack the extensive training required to be good, effective teachers (Campbell & Smith, 1997). Thus, in this chapter, we would like to provide an overview of several topics of specific interest to faculty relative to course design and establishing positive classroom climate. These topics constitute the foundation for our paradigm for learning wherein reflective teaching is centered on the learner, and active learning is a realized ideal.

Bloom's Taxonomy

Many (if not most) faculty have had the experience in which they design an assignment, collect student work, and then (while grading) bemoan the lack of "critical thinking" or "emotional maturity" students applied to their efforts. This is not a problem unique to contemporary faculty. Rather, this phenomenon was first formally addressed by an educational psychologist by the name of Benjamin Bloom almost 50 years ago. Realizing that teachers were at times ineffective at engaging students in rigorous learning activities, he created a series of three hierarchical domains to organize how students learn. These domains were specific to the following developmental categories of skills: cognitive, affective, and psychomotor (Bloom & Krathwohl, 1956). These hierarchical domains, together referred to as Bloom's Taxonomy, were created to explicitly describe what teachers should view as goals of the learning process and guide instructors to craft curricula that encouraged rigorous levels of thinking and learning across the board.

Bloom's Taxonomy is predicated on the notion that the interaction and overlap between the cognitive (knowledge and comprehension), affective (emotional reactions to various events/stimuli), and psychomotor (use of motor skills and physical coordination) domains can lead to higher level learning and balanced teaching (Bloom & Krathwohl, 1956). That said, when considering teaching at the university level, the domains representing cognitive and affective growth and development most often are focused upon, as they encompass both the notion of teaching content well (cognitive domain) and effectively interacting with others (affective domain) as the foundation for learning (Langan, 2010). This is illustrated by the EBE model proposed in Chapter 2. Thus, these are the focus of the remainder of this section.

Cognitive Domain

The cognitive domain was established to explain the acquisition of knowledge across a developmental trajectory. Within this domain, teachers are able to support the acquisition of higher level cognitive skills by accessing underlying principles of cognitive growth: complexity and consciousness (Maslovaty, Cohen, & Furman, 2008). The cognitive domain of Bloom's Taxonomy originally was described as containing six specific cognitive processes (knowledge, comprehension, application, analysis, synthesis, and evaluation), although these have been adapted in revisions of Bloom's Taxonomy. Each cognitive process is arranged in hierarchical order, with the lowest level cognitive skill (knowledge) developing first in students and the highest level cognitive skill (evaluation) emerging latest. Teaching that accesses skills characteristic of analysis, synthesis, and evaluation (the last three cognitive processes to develop) is considered to engage higher-level thinking and learning, even though these tend to be accessed least by teachers in classroom settings. The six original cognitive processes are briefly described in Figure 3–1 and are accompanied by descriptions of how teachers can set up experiences for students at each level of cognitive functioning.

Affective Domain

The affective domain explains the manner in which learners deal with emotional matters such as feelings, attitudes, and sources of motivation. This affective domain is structured to elicit behaviors on a continuum, from passive to autonomous, as students develop the ability to internalize affective aspects of learners (Maslovaty, Cohen, & Furman, 2008). As was the case with the cognitive domain, the affective domain of Bloom's Taxonomy contains specific processes,

	Description of Cognitive Processes	Access this Cognitive Process by:
Knowledge	Students demonstrating "knowledge" are able to recall information, define words, and demonstrate retrieval of information related to a topic.	Defining terms, describing items/actions, recalling information, answering basic yes/no and wh- questions
Comprehension	Students demonstrating "comprehension" are able to take in new information (through any modality) to encode new learning, reorder thoughts, and make predictions.	Summarizing ideas/concepts, comparing/contrasting ideas, outlining, demonstrating
Application	Students demonstrate "application" by using new knowledge to solve problems in a different way.	Developing alternate plans, articulating varied methods to study something, take different perspectives, planning/predicting outcomes for novel problems
Analysis	Students who demonstrate the use of "analysis" are able to view larger ideas as made up of smaller constituent parts. They can see patterns and organize information to determine relationships amongst elements and make inferences/generalizations.	Inferring information, prioritizing actions/needs, analyzing data, subdividing information to classify, and finding evidence to support hypotheses
Synthesis	Students who demonstrate "synthesis" can generate new knowledge by putting known elements together to form a whole new idea.	Modifying plots/plans, adapting plans to accept different parameters, elaborate on information, constructing new models, theorizing the answer to a problem
Evaluation	Students who demonstrate the use of "evaluation" can make judgments about the value of knowledge and can make choices based on reasoned arguments.	Presenting and defending opinions, assessing the value of a thought/idea, engaging in debates about a topic, making conclusions based on data

Figure 3–1. Bloom's Taxonomy: 6 Levels of the Cognitive Domain.

which describe the developmental acquisition of affective skills typical of learners. In the case of the affective domain, there are five processes that were placed in hierarchical order for use in encouraging higher-level learning. These include receiving, responding, valuing, organizing, and internalizing. The five processes of the affective domain are briefly described in Figure 3–2 with accompanying descriptions of how teachers can scaffold affective development in their students.

Is Bloom's Taxonomy the only framework for thinking about how students learn? Absolutely not. Many variations on learning

	Description of Affective Processes	Learners Demonstrate Affective Processes by:
Receiving	Students demonstrate "receiving" when they are passively attentive to various stimuli.	Listening with respect, being attentive
Responding	Students "responding" to stimuli are active participants who initially comply with requests but will eventually demonstrate a willingness to react/respond.	Asking questions, participating in class discussions, giving presentations
Valuing	"Valuing" is demonstrated when a learner determines the worth of an object, idea, or behavior and forms opinions to help with accepting or committing to this emergent internal understanding.	Valuing diversity, justifying behaviors, reporting issues/problems, forms opinions based on established social/academic mores
Organization	Students demonstrating "organization" can classify information into hierarchies of importance and can determine interrelationships. Students are able to adapt their behavior to their own emerging value systems.	Adhering to professional ethical standards, prioritizing/managing time effectively, accepting responsibility for own behavior
Internalizing	Students demonstrating "internalizing" behaviors are able to generalize their values into pervasive and predictable tendencies which control behavior. These values are integrated to form personal philosophies which consistently support interpersonal and intrapersonal interactions.	Cooperatively working with peers as part of a team, working independently in a responsible manner, objectively solve problems, changing opinions with advent of new evidence

Figure 3-2. Bloom's Taxonomy: 5 Levels of the Affective Domain.

taxonomies exist wherein developmental trajectories for learning are explained and described (e.g., Anderson & Krathwohl, 2001; Fink, 2003; Gagne &Briggs, 1974; Paul, 1993). These follow the same basic assumptions as did Bloom's Taxonomy: Learning occurs in a developmental progression and moves students from concrete to abstract thinking. We would argue, however, that the most worthwhile taxonomies to consider are those that address both cognitive and affective domains of learning, as it is in the intersection of these domains that meaningful learning happens. And, from our own experiences as teachers, we would agree with Fink's (2003) sentiment that when teachers and students reflect upon the process of learning, both groups of people want to drive learning past the point of simply understanding a concept; they want to apply it, as well.

Taking these notions and ideals into account, the issue depicted at the beginning of this section which asserted that many teachers have (at some point) been frustrated with a lack of critical thinking or emotional maturity in their student's work should be addressed. Some faculty might be hesitant to reflect critically on their own teaching practices as a potential cause of the frustrations they are experiencing. Yet we would argue that many times teaching is responsible for lack of student engagement or interest in a given subject. Thus, being able to carefully examine our pedagogical practices as teachers is really quite important. For those who adhere to the tenets and/or foundational underpinnings of Bloom's Taxonomy (or others), the solution to classroom frustrations is totally different and lies within the faculty members themselves. Perhaps the "problem" depicted wasn't with the students or their lack of critical thinking skills, but rather lay in how a course was designed or an assignment was conceived for students to complete. As noted in Chapter 1, Fink (2003, p. 3) asserts that despite having the desire for students to engage in higher-level thinking and learning, many faculty "continue to use a form of teaching that is not effective at promoting learning . . . rely[ing] heavily on lecturing as their main form of teaching" despite the fact that by itself, lecturing offers little support in helping students learns material in a meaningful way. Lecture alone rarely engages students in higher-level thinking and learning. Rather, faculty have the responsibility to provide instruction with rigor for their students in order to drive and encourage active learning at all levels of cognitive and affective development.

Bloom's Taxonomy is grounded in the assertion that if learning opportunities aren't designed to engage students in more critical forms of thinking and learning, students will not engage these higher level skills on their own. Rather, it is the responsibility of teachers to carefully craft learning opportunities to best facilitate high-level, high-quality learning in a manner that incorporates our own specialized content knowledge with our understanding of how to teach effectively, consistent with Shulman's notion of PCK described in Chapter 2. With this in mind, teachers who are able to adapt to affective characteristics of their students while simultaneously challenging them to ascend the cognitive hierarchy using instructional methods that are both rigorous and engaging are likely going to be effective instructors.

Learner-Centered Instruction

Taxonomies for learning are helpful, in part, because they help teachers conceptualize how learning happens. This is critically important, as we need to know how our students learn and how we can challenge them to attain higher levels of understanding within the courses we teach. That said, we would argue that it is not enough to simply use taxonomies to design learning opportunities within the context of traditional, lecture-based instructional settings. Rather, we would invoke the philosophies of Barr and Tagg (1995) with regard to learning and suggest that as teachers, faculty need to shift our efforts from "provid[ing] instruction" to "produc[ing] learning" (p. 697).

Barr and Tagg (1995) refer to this shift as being a change in paradigms, one that facilitates movement from traditional teaching (delivering instruction, covering predetermined course content, accessing curriculum in a linear manner) to learner-centered teaching wherein students are tasked actively with taking ownership for their learning while faculty facilitate and collaborate with students throughout this process. Why should faculty work to make this paradigm shift within their own classrooms? Why work to center our teaching on our students? Why have them take an active role in the learning process? Simply stated, traditional teaching is not enough. If traditional teaching simply means that we're offering courses, delivering lectures, and asking students to regurgitate information, we feel that too much potential is left behind, that our students miss out on important learning that can transcend the classroom setting. Consider the following charge:

> [As faculty, our] purpose is not to transfer knowledge but to create environments and experiences that bring students to discover and construct knowledge for themselves, to make students members of communities of learners that make discoveries and solve problems. [Faculty should aim] in fact, to create a series of ever more powerful learning environments. (Barr & Tagg, 1995, p. 699)

This is the heart of learner-centered teaching. It's the notion that our classrooms aren't (and shouldn't be) the end of a learning experience. Rather, it's our charge as faculty to engage students in learning that leads them to exploration and engagement beyond the scope of our syllabi. We strongly believe that teaching students to construct their own knowledge in ways meaningful and important on a personal level produces students who are learners beyond our courses.

An understanding of several key foundational concepts that underlie teaching for learning is helpful for faculty wishing to engage in learner-centered teaching. These concepts include constructivism, active learning, and reflective thinking. Each of these concepts will be discussed in detail in the following sections.

Active Learning as a Function of Constructivist Teaching

A quote often attributed to Socrates states that "education is the kindling of a flame, not the filling of a vessel." Constructivist teachers are those who adhere to this notion and strive to be facilitators of learning, rather than teachers who passively impart information to their students. To this end, our view of constructivist teaching is not a model of minimal guidance (Kirschner, Sweller, & Clark, 2006), but is a form of teaching in which students are able to actively seek out new forms of knowledge with the careful guidance and oversight of involved, facilitative faculty.

Defined broadly, constructivism is a theory of learning that allows students to construct their own knowledge and understanding of their world through considering past experiences, personal reflections, and existent world knowledge (Patton, 2002; Svinicki, 1999). Constructivists profess that the responsibility for learning lies with the learner while teachers guide students through the process of constructing meaning from their own realities (Crotty, 1998), assimilating new knowledge into their understanding of a particular topic or idea. Due to its emphasis on learner involvement in the process of acquiring knowledge, constructivism has served as the foundation for many successful instructional innovations particularly those involving active or cooperative learning (Svinicki, 1999).

Although constructivism itself is a theory of learning, active learning is one possible outcome of engaging in constructivist teaching. Inherent in the consideration of constructivist teaching is the need to make students "scholarly participants in the learning process" (Wrenn & Wrenn, 2009, p. 260) by promoting active learning experiences for all students (Gordon, 2009). Active learning is any

THE "LEARNER CENTERED-ACTIVE LEARNING" PARADIGM 49

instructional activity wherein students are able to broaden their knowledge base (learn) through active engagement with someone or something in an instructional setting (Prince, 2004). Some might consider active learning to be the intersection of thinking and doing, and they would be correct in this assumption.

Wrenn and Wrenn (2009, p. 259) characterize active learning as having the following characteristics:

- Students are not simply listening passively in the classroom environment; they are involved actively and are encouraged to participate.
- Teacher emphasis is not upon transmission of knowledge, but on students' development of skills.
- Students are involved in activities/practices, which promote higher order thinking (analysis, synthesis, evaluation).
- Students are engaged in activities such as reading, discussing, writing, or observing.
- Emphasis is placed on student exploration of their own ideals, beliefs, experience, and values.

Consistent with information presented earlier in this chapter, research also has demonstrated that in order for active learning to be effective, faculty must access affective aspects of a student's personality. What does this mean, and why is it an important consideration? Our experiences have led us to understand that if faculty are engaged in truly learner-centered teaching and are facilitating active learning, then a reciprocal relationship exists within the context of our classrooms that cannot be ignored. To encourage students to be open to new and different learning opportunities and be risk takers as learners, faculty build trusting relationships by treating students as individuals with inherent value, deserving of respect. Considering the affective needs of our students demonstrates our willingness, as faculty, to acknowledge that students are important partners in the learning process. To this end, Wrenn & Wrenn provided several important behaviors faculty can adopt to support student learning by accessing affective aspects of their personalities (p. 260):

- Demonstrate an interest in students as unique individuals.
- Acknowledge students' attitudes/feelings related to a class, assignment, etc.

- Encourage students to seek answers to their questions.
- Provide explicit communication related to the importance of learning and why it's important to the task at hand.
- Encourage students to independently form their own viewpoints and opinions to support and inform learning.

Overall, active learning is considered to be an effective teaching practice, one that has proven effectiveness in improving student attitudes, developing skills to apply new knowledge to novel situations, improving written skills, retaining material, motivating students, and developing thinking skills (Bonwell & Eison, 1991; Fink, 2003; McKeachie, 1999; Prince, 2004).

Active Learning in Practice

For faculty teaching future speech-language pathologists and/or audiologists, active learning strategies provide an opportunity for students to solve problems as involved participants, whether individually or in groups of students. To demonstrate this, a comparison of traditional, lecture-based instruction to active learning highlights the important differences between these opposing teaching strategies.

Suppose that you were preparing to teach a class about anatomy and physiology, with specific attention paid to the structures critical for communication in the brain. In a traditional lecture setting, a teacher might prepare a PowerPoint presentation with photographs and diagrams to indicate the arrangement and visual appearance of each critical structure. Important points would be noted on each slide, with bulleted points spelling out the most important information for students to know. Students passively take notes, ask questions for clarification, and endeavor to comprehend a topic that is relatively unknown to them.

Alternatively, active learning techniques might incorporate just a few PowerPoint slides, used to frame topics for group discussion. Students are broken into collaborative groups and are asked to work together to reconstruct models of each lobe of the brain, paying special attention to communication-related structures. During the first half of class, students construct their three-dimensional lobes of the brain and are then asked to share their creations with the class, explaining their model, the surrounding structures, and the importance of each structure for communication.

These exemplar classes both meet criteria for addressing relevant course content, but very different methods were used to foster learning. Which method encouraged the highest levels of thinking and learning? The traditional method asked students to display the processes of knowledge and comprehension, the two lowest levels of the cognitive domain within Bloom's Taxonomy. In contrast, the active learning model accessed the processes of analysis and synthesis to complete the in-class activity. In this example, active-learning strategies led to the facilitation of higher levels of thinking and problem solving, an outcome desirable to most faculty today (Fink, 2003).

This example constitutes just one instance of how active learning techniques can be integrated into a classroom environment. Chapter 6 highlights a variety of other active learning techniques and provides illustrative examples of how these techniques can be implemented by faculty within a variety of classes.

Reflective Thinking and Learning as a Philosophy

Predominantly, active reflection that takes place in educational settings is completed by faculty, rather than students, though this is not necessarily appropriate (Griffiths, 2010). As faculty, we strive to encourage a deeper processing of information to ensure that our students not only understand information disseminated during class time, but that they consider it critically, as well. This process is referred to as reflective learning and was described by Schön (1983) as a process that necessitates the examination of a learner's values, beliefs, and emotions. Boyd and Fales (1983) expanded upon this notion to define reflective learning by saying:

> The process of reflection is the core difference between whether a person repeats the same experience several times becoming highly proficient at one behavior, or learns from experience in such a way that he or she is cognitively or affectively changed. (p. 100)

Although students themselves are engaged in reflective learning, it is us, as faculty, who act to facilitate this reflection. In fact, fostering these reflective skills in our students is time well spent in the classroom, as most college students lack the metacognitive awareness of how reflection can function as an aid to learning and must be directly taught these skills (Boyd & Fales, 1983). The good news is, reflective learning can be taught directly to students, and long-term benefits can be realized from the teaching of these skills (Griffiths, 2010). Generally speaking, research would suggest that faculty be explicit in their talking about reflection with students, making them aware of what reflection is and how it can be used as to compliment low-level cognitive processes to engage in higher-level critical thinking. And, beyond the classroom environment, the added value of spending time teaching about reflection is that we then can expect generalization of these reflective skills as our students adapt to their responsibilities as student clinicians. Thus, teaching about reflection not only supports students in their classroom learning, but in their clinical practice, as well.

So what might reflective learning look like in a classroom environment? Reflective learning techniques can be used in conjunction with virtually any aspect of a given course and can include journaling, analysis of case studies, peer evaluations, blogging, peer teaching, or any other activity that asks that students analyze, review, reconstruct, or edit their own work or the work of their peers (Brockbank & McGill, 2007). As an example, consider a faculty member teaching graduate students about collecting language samples and completing a subsequent transcription and analysis of all utterances collected. In class, this teacher might well cover the ins and outs of language sample collection and might instruct students about the efficacy of and process inherent in language sample analysis. Reflective learning easily could be made an integral part of this experience for students in a variety of ways:

- Students could be asked to write a reflective paper about their performance as clinicians collecting their first language samples, making certain to highlight positive and negative aspects of their clinical experiences and suggesting how to improve or maintain various levels of performance.
- Students could evaluate the final reports written by their peers, looking specifically at form and content.

- Based on their experiences with the language sample collection/analysis project, students could be asked to draft a list of preferred language sample collection techniques to be shared with future graduate students or undergraduates in their department.

As was the case with active learning techniques, the application of reflective learning activities is limited by only the creativity and ingenuity of the faculty member looking to make changes to his/her classroom environment.

Concluding Thoughts

In sum, while taxonomies, constructivist principles, and reflective learning might seem like a mismatched combination of educationally related concepts, they really are not. These main themes from Chapter 3 all have one very important commonality: They focus on faculty as facilitators of learning, rather than *deliverers* of information. This is a critical difference, both in theory and in practice. We want to encourage active and reflective learning in order to encourage student engagement and learning that extends beyond our immediate classroom environment. As involved participants in learning, students accept responsibility for being part of the classroom discourse and take on the role of a participant in their educational process, rather than assuming the role of a passive recipient. This, in turn, fosters the development of higher-level critical thinking skills, which allow students to consider course content in ways not possible in more traditional, passive learning environments. Simply stated, this constitutes our shared vision for teachers and students in higher education: active, reflective involvement for all who are stakeholders in the process.

This book was conceived to focus CSD faculty on the importance of SOTL and EBE to improve our practice as teachers. For, much as we teach our students to be clinicians who practice in a manner supported by evidence, we should do that same as professional educators. Thus, set the stage for you to explore these concepts and consider them in light of your own classroom (and nonclassroom) experiences. Chapters 4, 5, 6, and 7 of this text will introduce the next steps that follow our initial discussion of what we consider to be the foundational aspects of teaching: evidence-based methods of putting our learner-centered teaching philosophy into action, with in-depth suggestions for faculty related to course design, classroom communication, student engagement, and assessing learning.

References

Anderson, L., & Krathwohl, D. (Eds.). (2001). *A taxonomy for learning, teaching, and assessing: A revision of bloom's taxonomy of educational objectives*. Boston, MA: Allyn & Bacon.

Barr, R., & Tagg, J. (1995). From teaching to learning: A new paradigm for undergraduate education. *Change, 27*(6), 697–710.

Bloom, B., & Krathwohl, D. (1956). *Taxonomy of educational objectives: The classification of educational goals*. New York, NY: Longmans, Green, Co.

Bonwell, C., & Eison, J. (1991). *Active Learning: Creating Excitement in the Classroom AEHE-ERIC Higher Education Report No. 1*. Washington, DC: Jossey-Bass.

Boyd, E., & Fales, A. (1983). Reflective learning: Key to learning from experience. *Journal of Humanistic Psychology, 23*(2), 99–117.

Brockbank, A., & McGill, I. (2007). *Facilitating reflective learning in higher education* (2nd ed.). New York, NY: McGraw-Hill.

Campbell, W., & Smith, K. (1997). *New paradigms for college teaching*. Edina, MN: Interaction Book.

Crotty, M. (1998). *The foundations of social research: Meaning and perspective in the research process*. London, UK: Sage.

Fink, L. (2003). *Creating significant learning experiences: An integrated approach to designing college courses*. San Francisco, CA: Jossey-Bass.

Gagne, R., & Briggs, L. (1974). *Principles of instructional design* (2nd ed.). Austin, TX: Hold, Rinehart, and Winston.

Gordon, M. (2009). Toward a pragmatic discourse on constructivism: Reflection on lessons from practice. *Educational Studies, 45*, 39–58.

Griffiths, E. (2010). Clearing the misty landscape: Teaching students what they didn't know then, but know now. *College Teaching, 58*, 32–37.

Kirschner, P., Sweller, J., & Clark, R. (2006). Why minimal guidance during instruction does not work: An analysis or the failure of constructivist, discovery, problem-based, experiential, and inquiry-based teaching. *Educational Psychologist, 41*(2), 75–86.

Langan, T. (2010). *Bloom's taxonomy for affective learning and teaching.* Retrieved from http://www.wisc-online.com/objects/viewObject.aspx?ID=OTT402

Marzano, R., & Kendall, J. (2007). *The new taxonomy of educational objectives* (2nd ed.). Thousand Oaks, CA: Corwin Press.

Maslovaty, N., Cohen, A., & Furman, S. (2008). The structural validity of the "ideal student" multi-faceted theory among education students. *Studies in Educational Evaluation, 34*(3), 165–172.

McKeachie, W. (1999). *Teaching tips: Strategies, research and theory for college and university teachers* (10th ed.). Boston, MA: Houghton Mifflin.

Patton, M. (2002). *Qualitative research and evaluation methods* (3rd ed.). Thousand Oaks, CA: Sage.

Paul, R. (1993). *Critical thinking: How to prepare student for a rapidly changing world.* Santa Rosa, CA: The Foundation for Critical Thinking.

Prince, M. (2004). Does active learning work? A review of the research. *Journal of Engineering Education, 93*(3), 223–231.

Schön, D. (1983). *The reflective practitioner: How professionals think in action.* New York, NY: Basic Books.

Shulman, L. (2002). Making differences: A table of learning change. *Change, 34*(6), 36–45.

Svinicki, M. (1999). New directions in learning and motivation. In M. D. Svinicki (Ed.), *Teaching and Learning on the edge of the millennium: Building on what we have learned.* San Francisco, CA: Jossey-Bass.

Wrenn, J. & Wrenn, B. (2009). Enchancing learning by integrating theory and practice. *International Journal of Teaching and Learning in Higher Education, 21*(2), 258–268.

4

Before You Teach: Course Design and Preparation

> *We can best decide, as guides, what "sites" to have our student "tourists" visit and what specific "culture" they should experience in their brief time there only if we are clear about the particular understandings about the culture we want them to take home.*
> —Wiggins and McTighe, 2005, p. 15

As you reflect on your teaching, perhaps you'll find that you want to incorporate EBE into your courses and, in doing so, create a course that actively engages your students with the course content. Perhaps you will endeavor to move from being a good teacher to a scholarly teacher and eventually to incorporating the scholarship of teaching and learning (SOTL) into some or all of your courses (see Chapter 1). In addition, you might decide to utilize learner-centered instruction and active learning principles (see Chapter 3) into your courses. However, in order for you to do this, you will need to design, redesign, or at the very least, tweak your course. It also means that you will need to dedicate a good deal of time and energy to the process. In addition, as Childre, Sands, and Pope (2009) state, it "requires a paradigm shift in which textbooks are one of a variety of teaching tools rather than the sole basis for daily teaching" (p. 6). Therefore, you will not be able to just open the textbook you ordered for the course and list off the chapters on your syllabus, nor will you be able to continue to use your lecture notes that are 15 years old. However, before you panic, remember that the time that you invest up-front in designing the course will pay off in more active student engagement and improved learning outcomes. This chapter reviews the use of backward design (Wiggins & McTighe, 1998, 2005) and creating significant learning (Fink, 2003) as methods to use as you design and prepare your new and improved course. The chapter provides you with the evidence available regarding their effectiveness and examples of how these concepts can be implemented in courses.

Backward Design

One approach to course design is the use of backward design, which was proposed by Wiggins and McTighe in 1998 and revised in 2005. Backward design argues "that you cannot plan how you're going to teach until you know exactly what you want your students to learn" (Childre et al., 2009, p. 7). Backward design is a guide for instructors, which provides instructors with the steps for determining what students should know and understand, how it will be evaluated, and then how it will be taught. The three stages of backward design include identifying desired results, determining acceptable evidence, and planning learning experiences and instruction.

Stage 1: Identify Desired Results

Identifying desired results means that we start our course design process by determining what our students should know, understand, or be able to do by the end of the course. Or, as Wiggins and McTighe (2005) put it, we must identify "what *enduring* understandings are desired?" (p.17). To answer this question, we need to examine our learner outcomes, the American Speech-Language-Hearing Association's (ASHA) knowledge and skills acquisition (KASA) standards in speech-language pathology (SLP) (ASHA, 2009a) or audiology (ASHA, 2009b), and curricular expectations within our specific program and/or institution. We also need to determine what information is worth being familiar with versus information that is important to actually know or what skills are important to be able to do versus what concepts are critical to know or represent "enduring understanding." For example, do you expect your SLP students to know how to do auditory evoked potential (AEP) measurements, or is it all right for them to be familiar with AEPs and the information obtained from this assessment? What depth of understanding do you expect undergraduate communication disorders students to have with regards to dysphagia or augmentative and alternative communication (AAC) devices? Or what are your clinical expectations for a first semester graduate student versus a fourth semester graduate student?

An additional aspect to consider when we are identifying the desired results for our student is the six facets of understanding: explanation, interpretation, application, perspective, empathy, and self-knowledge (Wiggins & McTighe, 2005). The six facets of understanding are similar to Bloom's taxonomy (Bloom & Krathwohl, 1956) (see Chapter 3). In either case, we need to consider the desired results of our course in relationship to what we are asking our students to be able to do. Do we want the students to explain the difference between syntax and pragmatics, speech-language pathology and audiology? Or do we expect our students to apply their knowledge of language development to breakdowns in language due to a specified language disorder? After we have established or clarified the desired outcomes or the curricular priorities of the course, we then are able to move on to the next stage in the course design process.

Stage 2: Determine Acceptable Evidence

According to Wiggins and McTighe (2005), stage 2 in the backward design approach takes the curricular priorities and determines what evidence would be considered acceptable in demonstrating that the students have met the desired results. This means that, instead of designing the course based on what content will be covered, the course is designed based on what evidence will be needed to determine that the learning outcomes for the course have been met. This evidence can be formal and informal assessment that takes place throughout the course. Specifically, four types of evidence should be reviewed: performance tasks, academic prompts, quiz and test items, and informal checks of understanding. Performance tasks are complex assignments that present the student with a real-life issue or problem that they may be likely to encounter as an adult. The tasks may be short-term tasks, long-term tasks, and/or tasks that can be done in several stages or steps. For example, the performance task could be that students are presented with a hypothetical patient whom they might encounter in the clinical setting and are asked to identify the areas that would need to be assessed during their diagnostic evaluation. Another task might be to ask students to listen to an audio sample and phonetically transcribe the single word productions of a child with a speech sound disorder.

Academic prompts require students to produce a specific academic product (i.e., paper, performance) based on an open-ended question. It requires a student to critically evaluate information and to apply it to the specific academic problem. The problems or questions used in academic prompts typically are "only asked of students in school" (Wiggins & McTighe, 2005, p. 153). Therefore, they differ from performance tasks in that performance tasks could be encountered by an individual within the course of his or her daily life, whereas an academic prompt is a question or problem that typically is confined to a classroom setting. An example of an academic prompt may be to create a PowerPoint presentation that lists and explains the possible causes of conductive hearing loss in an adult; or writing the vowels in on the vowel quadrilateral; or writing a paper about a specified language disorder.

The third and most frequently used type of evidence in the academic setting is a quiz or test item. Test and quiz items assess the student's knowledge and understanding of factual information or concepts or the demonstration of a specific skill(s) (see Chapter 7 for more information regarding assessment).

Finally, informal checks of understanding are an ongoing form of classroom assessment in which the instructor observes student interaction with the material, asks questions during the class, or examines students' work to determine the level of understanding of the course concepts. These informal checks of understanding or formative forms of assessment are not linked to grades, but rather are a check for the instructor as to the students' understanding of the course concepts. For example, informal checks may include an in-class assignment, asking students questions during class, minute papers (see Chapter 7), or having students write what they learned in the class that day or what questions they have regarding the concepts being discussed. These informal checks enable the instructor to make changes to the both the content being covered and the manner in which the content is being covered at that point in the class. Therefore, if the instructor determines that some confusion exists regarding the course material that day, the instructor may provide the class with additional examples of the concepts, or repeat the material in a different format. On the other hand, if the instructor determines that the students really understand the material, then the instructor will move on to new material based on that feedback.

Stage 3: Plan Learning Experiences and Instruction

The third and final stage in the backward design process is planning the learning experiences and instruction to accompany the end results specified in the first two steps of the design process (Wiggins & McTighe, 2005). Therefore, after you have identified what evidence is needed to say that the learning outcomes have been met, you then can plan the most appropriate learning experiences that will be used to meet the learning outcomes and provide you with evidence needed to demonstrate the knowledge obtained. (Chapter 6 provides several specific examples of active learning tasks that can be utilized.)

In this stage, the instructor needs to make decisions regarding the pedagogical methods being used, the sequence of the information and activities for the course, and the resources needed to meet the learning outcomes and assessment evidence. Instructors, therefore, need to ask themselves the following questions (Wiggins & McTighe, 2005):

- What knowledge—facts, concepts, or principles—will the students need in order to meet the desired learner outcomes for the course?

- What skills—process, procedures, or strategies—will the students need?
- What activities can be utilized to provide the students with the knowledge and/or skills?
- What will directly be taught to the students?
- What will be mentored through active learning tasks?
- What materials and resources can be utilized to meet the course goals?

The instructor must continually balance knowledge and skill acquisition with the means of assessment or what evidence will be obtained in order to determine whether the learning outcome has been met.

Wiggins and McTighe (2005) recommend the use of "WHERETO" as a method for planning engaging and effective learning experiences. WHERETO includes the following elements:

Where is it going?

Hook the students

Explore and equip

Rethink and revise

Exhibit and evaluate

Tailor to student needs, interests, and styles

Organize for maximum engagement and effectiveness. (p. 147)

Thus, "where is it going" asks the instructor to have clear goals or learner outcomes with a rationale for them. It requires the instructor to know where the students are coming from with regard to their prior knowledge, skills, experiences, and learning style. In addition, the work within the course needs to be purposeful not only from the instructor's viewpoint, but also from the student's perspective.

Hooking the students requires the instructor to engage the students by asking questions, providing insights into problems, presenting challenging problems, or providing anecdotes (Wiggins & McTighe, 2005). To engage students, the instructor needs to pique their intellectual interests and hold them throughout the course. Wiggins and McTighe suggest the following conditions can be used to achieve this: "instant immersion in questions, problems, challenges, situations or stories that require the student's wits, not just school knowledge" (p. 207); "thought provocations" (p. 207); "experiential shocks" (p. 207); "personal shock" (p. 207); "differing points of view or multiple perspectives on an issue" (p. 208).

To explore and equip students, the instructor needs to create experiences that will provide the students with the knowledge, skills, and experiences to meet the learning outcomes (Wiggins & McTighe, 2005). The students will explore the content and/or skills for the course through a variety of well-designed experiences created by the instructor. Further, the instructor will equip the students with the tools necessary to perform the specific skills needed to meet the learning outcomes.

According to Wiggins and McTighe (2005), as instructors are planning the course, they need to intentionally provide the students with a variety of opportunities that will enable them to rethink the major concepts of the course. Students also need to have the opportunity to reflect on their learning of the course concepts and to revise their work, as needed. The creation of activities or opportunities for the students to rethink, revise, and reflect on the course material should lead to a greater depth of understanding of the course concepts.

The next element in the plan is to exhibit and evaluate. Here activities are designed to enable students to self-assess, self-evaluate, and make adjustments individually and as a group (Wiggins & McTighe, 2005). Students need to learn to honestly assess their own understanding of information and to make adjustments in their learning. The instructor needs to create specific ongoing opportunities for students to engage in self-assessment as it helps to develop life-long learning skills.

In general, the instructor needs to tailor and personalize the course in order to meet the needs of the students (Wiggins & McTighe, 2005). To do this, the instructor needs to examine the learning styles of the students, prior knowledge, student interests, and individual student needs. When examining individual student needs and interests, it is important to differentiate learning based on the content being learned, the processes by which the content is being learned, and the variety of products that can be used to demonstrate the knowledge. The goal of tailoring the course for the students is to maximize student engagement and to create a course that is effective for all of the students to learn and demonstrate the knowledge and skills being taught.

The final element of planning is organizing for optimal effectiveness (Wiggins & McTighe, 2005). At this point, all of the previous elements are examined to determine the best sequence for not only teaching the course content, but for students to learn the information. The sequence of the information should reflect "a constant movement back and forth between whole–part–whole and learning–doing–reflecting" (Wiggins & McTighe, 2005, p. 220).

So now you have reached the end of the process of backward design. You have identified the desired results, determined the acceptable evidence, and planned the learning experiences and instruction. However, if the goal is to engage in EBE, then prior to implementing the backward design approach (Wiggins & McTighe, 2005), we need to examine the available research in the scholarship of teaching and learning (SOTL).

Evidence for Backward Design

Childre and colleagues (2009) provide anecdotal evidence supporting the use of backward design. Specifically, they state that, "through the use of the backward design approach, learning can become relevant and meaningful for all students, supporting their mastery of general curricular standards. When standards, assessment, and inquiry-oriented activities drive the curriculum, learning can be transformed" (Childre, et al., 2009, p. 14). In addition, Fink (2003) utilizes aspects of backward design as he presents his model for creating significant learning. More recently, Wiggins and McTighe (2007) have taken the concepts and success that they have had with backward design and applied them to the overall school setting and curriculum design. *Schooling by Design* recommends working backward in rebuilding the curriculum of our schools by starting with the mission and then moving backward through curriculum and assessment; principles of learning and instructional design; implementing structures, policies, practices, and resources that are consistent with the mission; incorporating feedback and adjustment within the system; and ending with meeting the desired results (Wiggins & McTighe, 2007). Therefore, some anecdotal evidence exists for the use of backward design; however, in our review of the literature, we were unable to find any quantitative evidence that evaluates this approach.

Applying Backward Design: A Practice Example

Now that you have the general theoretical concepts of backward design and you are aware that only limited anecdotal evidence exists to support its use, what would it look like in a communication disorders course? Let's say that you have been scheduled to teach an undergraduate level course in phonetics and phonology. The students in this course are freshman and sophomore communication disorders majors, who have taken an introductory course in communication disorders. Vignette 4–1 provides a brief overview of the thought process involved in utilizing backward design for this course.

Creating Significant Learning

In 2003, L. Dee Fink wrote *Creating Significant Learning Experiences: An Integrated Approach to Designing College Courses*, in which he builds on Bloom's taxonomy (Bloom & Krathwohl, 1956) and Wiggins and McTighe's (1998) six facets of understanding. Fink recommended a new taxonomy of learning that emphasized six interacting dimensions of learning: foundational knowledge, application, integration, human dimension, caring, and learning how to learn (Table 4–1). In designing an integrated course, Fink (2003, 2004) proposed three phases that began with building strong primary components, assembling the components into a coherent whole, and concluding with finishing the important remaining tasks. The following section provides a brief overview of Fink's concepts and examples of how they can be applied to courses in the fields of communication sciences and disorders.

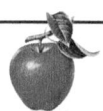

Vignette 4–1. Application of Backward Design: Phonetics and Phonology

Stage 1—Identifying Desired Results	Stage 2—Determine Acceptable Evidence		Stage 3—Planning the Learning Experiences and Instruction
	Performance Tasks or Projects—Rubric item scores on tasks/projects	Other Evidence	
Phonetic transcription of normal and disordered speech	• Accurate transcription of normal conversational speech • Accurate transcription of disordered conversational speech	• Homework assignments • Tests / quizzes • Minute papers	• Teach phonetic transcription • Listening exercises of typical and disordered speech samples
Knowledge and understanding of place-manner-voice of consonants	Able to explain errors in production of consonants based on place-manner-voicing	• Homework assignments • Tests/quizzes • Minute papers	• Teach phonetic transcription of consonants • Worksheets used to organize information
Knowledge and understanding of height, advancement, round, and tense/lax for vowels	Able to explain errors in production of vowels based on tongue height, advancement, rounding, and tense/lax	• Homework assignments • Tests/quizzes • Minute papers	• Teach phonetic transcription of vowels • Worksheets used to organize information
Phonological processes/patterns	Accurate analysis of phonological processes/patterns	• Homework assignments • Tests/quizzes • Minute papers	• Teach phonological processes • Practice applying knowledge in various activities

Table 4–1. Bloom's Taxonomy (Bloom & Krathwohl, 1956), Wiggins and McTighe's (1998; 2005) Six Facets of Understanding, and Fink's (2003) Six Interacting Dimensions of Learning

Bloom's Taxonomy—Traditional (Cognitive) Content-Centered Learning Taxonomy (Bloom & Krathwohl, 1956)

Knowledge—recognizes and recalls facts and specifics

Comprehension—interprets, translates, summaries, or paraphrases information

Application—uses information in a situation different from original learning context

Analysis—separates whole into parts until relationship among elements is clear

Synthesis—combines elements to form new entity from original ones

Evaluation—involves acts of decision making, judging, or selecting based on criteria and rational

Wiggins & McTighe (2005) Six Facets of Understanding (p. 343)

Explanation—provides thorough, supported, and justifiable accounts of phenomena, facts, and data

Interpretation—tells meaningful stories; offers apt translations; provides a revealing historical or personal dimension to ideas and events; makes something personal or accessible through images, anecdotes, analogies, or models

Application—effectively uses and adapts knowledge in diverse contexts

Perspective—sees points of view, with critical eyes and eats; sees the big picture

Empathy—gets inside, finds value in what others might find odd, alien, or implausible; perceives sensitively, based on prior direct experience

Self-knowledge—perceives the personal style, prejudices, projections, and habits or mind that both shape and impede understanding; be aware of what is not understood and why it is so hard to understand

continues

Table 4–1. *continued*

Fink's (2003, p. 30–32) Six Interacting Dimensions of Learning
Foundational knowledge—describes understanding and remembering specific information and ideas
Application—learning how to engaging in some new type of intellectual, physical, or social action
Integration—involves connecting learned material with other ideas, people or realms of life
Human dimension—learning important information about oneself or others
Caring—developing new feelings, interests, and values
Learning how to learn—becoming a better student by learning to be inquisitive and self-directed

Initial Design Phase: Building Strong Primary Components

Identifying Situational Factors

Using Fink's (2003) approach to course design begins with identifying the important situational factors that may impact or influence the course. The situational factors include the specific context of the teaching and learning situation, such as, number of students in the class, course level, length of class time, and frequency of class meeting times, and whether the class will be taught in an online, classroom setting, or a combination of formats. Many of these are elements of the teacher-learner interaction, which were discussed in Chapter 2. Another situational factor is the expectations of external groups, including the department, institution, profession, and society. Thus, considering issues such as whether the introduction to communication disorders class is required by other departments on campus or examining ASHA's KASA summary form to ensure that the courses provide the students with the appropriate information to meet the standards. A third situational factor to consider when designing your course is the nature of the subject. This would include determining whether the course subject matter is convergent or has a single correct answer versus divergent or has multiple solutions or perspectives to the problem, the knowledge and/or skills required for the subject matter, and the stability of the course content. From there, the instructor should consider the characteristics of the learners; including their life situations; life and professional goals; reasons for enrolling in the course; prior experiences, knowledge, and attitudes regarding the subject; and the learning styles of the students. In addition to examining the student's characteristics, the instructor also needs to examine his or her own characteristics as a teacher. These characteristics could include whether you have had previous experience teaching the course; your knowledge, skills, and attitudes regarding the course and the process of teaching; and your level of confidence and competence with teaching the course material. The final situational factor to consider is whether any special pedagogical challenges exist for this course. Pedagogical challenges could include students' fear of research as they enter your research methods course or their belief that the only childhood language disorder they need to know about is autism and that they already know everything there is about this subject.

If the elements that Fink describes as situational factors sound familiar, it is because they overlap with elements of the evidence-based education (EBE) model presented in Chapter 2. Specifically, Fink's situational factors overlap with both the teacher-learner interaction elements and pedagogical content knowledge (PCK) (discussed in Chapters 1 and 2). Therefore, in the initial stage of creating significant learning in your course you need to begin to implement the elements of EBE: PCK and teacher-learner interaction.

Learning Goals

After the situational factors have been identified, the instructor utilizes a backward design, proposed by Wiggins and McTighe (2005), to determine the learning goals for the course and the feedback and assessment procedures for determining whether the learning goals have been obtained. In determining the learning goals, Fink (2003) emphasizes six interacting dimensions of learning: foundational knowledge, application, integration, human dimension, caring, and learning how to learn. *Foundational knowledge* encompasses the key information, facts, terms, formula, concepts, and relationships that are important for students to understand and remember as they progress both academically and professionally within the field. For example, foundational knowledge concepts in communication disorders would include knowledge of the differences between the professions of speech-language pathology and audiology; terms such as syntax, phonology, morphology, semantics, pragmatics, conductive-hearing loss, sensorineural hearing loss, repetitions, prolongations, and so on; formulas for calculating MLU or TTR; and relationships such as relationships between speech, language, and communication, or the components of speech or language, or the relationship between sound traveling and the parts of the ear.

The learning dimension of *application* asks the instructor to consider what kinds of thinking (i.e., critical thinking, creative thinking, or practical thinking), skills, and complex projects are important for the student to learn. Examples of the learning dimension within the fields of communication sciences and disorders could include phonetic transcription of disordered speech, pure-tone audiometry testing, critical analysis of research studies, analysis of language samples, and the examination of diagnostic test scores in determining the need for intervention.

The instructor also needs to determine what connections the students need to make between the course ideas, information, and their own personal and social lives. This is the learning dimension of *integration*. Some general ways to incorporate integration tasks into your course are through case studies, essay questions in which students are asked to explain connections between concepts, or tasks that require the students to explain the relevance of an article in the newspaper or popular press. Therefore, the tasks could include providing students with a newspaper article regarding the use of cochlear implants in hearing-impaired children; asking students to develop a presentation for elementary school teachers in which they help teachers understand when to refer children for services and ways to incorporate language tasks into the classroom setting; or explaining to their own family members intervention options for either an adult or child family member with a communication disorder.

The fourth dimension is the *human dimension*, which enables students to discover "how to interact more effectively with oneself and with others" (Fink, 2003, p. 74). Thus, we are asking our students to examine their own ideas, perceptions, and interactions along with other individual's ideas, perceptions, and interactions in order to improve their understanding of themselves and others. One way to incorporate the human dimension into your course is by having students take a survey in which they are to asked to respond (on a Likert scale from strongly agree to strongly disagree) to statements regarding their own strengths and challenges in the treatment and/or assessment of various communication disorders; write reflections on their strengths and challenges with the assessment of fluency or voice disorders; or write reflections on their clinical development from one semester to the next. All of these are examples of how the human dimension can be built into communication disorders courses.

From there, the instructor needs to determine whether, as a result of the course, the students are expected to demonstrate changes in their feelings, interests, or values. This aspect of learning represents the *caring* dimension, and it is assumed that when students care more about a topic, then they will be more willing to learn about the topic. Given the caring nature of the disciplines of communication disorders, this dimension should be rather easy to integrate into a course. For example, students could be asked to keep a log or journal regarding their level of interest and caring regarding topics taught in class or their level of interest and caring about the patients they work with in the clinical setting. Students also could be asked to complete a survey at the beginning and end of the semester that asks questions about their appreciation of the importance of the discipline in impacting the lives of others.

The final learning dimension proposed by Fink is *learning how to learn*. Do you want your students to learn how to be good students? Engage in inquiry and construct knowledge with the material? Become self-directed learners in this content area? Some ways to integrate learning how to learn into your communication disorders course include using a survey in a research methods course in which students are asked the best ways to locate information on specific topics; having students reflect on the learning activities over the course of the semester and discuss the strengths and challenges of learning for them by each of the methods; having students rate their comfort level with professional resources utilized in the clinical setting; or having students explain why certain sources of information are more or less trustworthy.

In summary, as the instructor develops a course, he or she needs to determine the learning goals for the course, and these learning goals should cover all six dimensions of learning. Therefore, the instructor should have learning goals for foundational knowledge, application, integration, the human dimension, caring, and learning how to learn developed into each course.

Feedback and Assessment

When the learning goals for each learning dimension have been determined, the next step in the initial phase of course design is to determine the feedback and assessment measures. Fink (2003) recommends that we expand our "view of feedback and assessment to include more *educative* assessment" (p. 82). The ultimate goal of assessment is to support learning. (See Chapter 7 with regard to specific types and styles of assessment that could be utilized within your courses.) As we examine the feedback and assessment that we will be using within our courses, we should make sure that we are meeting the goal of supporting all six dimensions of learning, as well as providing more authentic grading. This can be accomplished through educative assessment, which has "four primary components: forward-looking assessment, criteria and standards, self-assessment, and 'FIDeLity' feedback" (Fink, 2003, p. 83). In forward-looking assessment, we create real-life assignments (e.g., questions, exercises, problems, class discussions, etc.) that require the students to utilize the information learned. These assignments should engage the students in situations in which they are likely to find themselves where they would need to apply or incorporate the concepts that they have learned in the course. Therefore, instead of giving the students a quiz or exam that asks them to give back information that they have been taught, the students are asked to apply the information to a potential real-world situation, which typically would require an individual to utilize the information learned from the course. One easy example that we can make use of in our courses is case studies. Presenting students with a specific case, whether real or specifically created for the class, requires that students make use of information from the class to answer specific questions about the case. Another way to present students with real-life experiences is by utilizing YouTube videos that present the everyday person with a communication disorder. For example, in a fluency disorders course, students could be asked to view specified YouTube videos, transcribe the speech sample, and analyze the core behaviors, secondary behaviors, and feelings and attitudes of the person on the video.

As part of determining the feedback and assessment procedures for a course, the instructor needs to thoroughly and clearly explain the criteria and standards that will used to assess the students' work. The criteria and standards should be specific so that the student knows what would constitute a poor, fair, good, or exceptional example of the assigned task or activity. The criteria and standards may be specific KASA criteria and standards in which the specific program determines the required level of success that needs to be met to progress. On the other hand, the criteria could be the level of accuracy that a student needs to obtain when transcribing a language sample, calculating percent of dysfluent utterances in an individual's speech or their MLU; or the level of accuracy a student needs to meet when calibrating a hearing aid for a specific hearing loss.

In addition to the instructor assessing the students' progress on the learning outcomes, students should also be asked to assess their own perception of their progress. By creating multiple opportunities for students to self-assess, we also are teaching the students to be self-directed learners, a skill that is needed later in life when their employer or supervisor asks them to assess their own performance. This self-assessment can take many forms including grading their own performance on an assignment prior to handing the assignment in for the instructor to assess; students' assessment of each other's work; assessment of other student's work and then assessing their own work; or students' assessment of their own work and comparing it to the instructor's assessment of the work, which is followed by the student making changes in the work based on the assessment.

The fourth and final feature of feedback and assessment is FIDeLity feedback or good feedback. Fink (2003) defines FIDeLity as feedback that is *Frequent*—occurring at least weekly; *Immediate*—occurring preferably during the class when the learning activity is done; *Discriminating* in that it is based on the standards and criteria; and done *Lovingly* and supportively, which helps to get the feedback through to the student.

Teaching and Learning Activities

At this point in the course design or redesign, you have examined the situational factors that may play a role in the course, determined the learning goals for the course, and determined the feedback and assessment measures that you will use. The next step is to design the teaching and learning activities, which means that you need to determine what the students will be doing in the course to be successful on the feedback and assessment activities and meet the learning goals for the course. Fink (2003) suggests the use of active learning tasks. (See Chapter 6 for specific examples of active learning tasks that can be utilized to engage students in your courses.) He takes a holistic view of active learning that incorporates three components: information and ideas, experiences, and reflective dialogue. Therefore, as you decide what teaching and learning activities that you will incorporate in a course, you should attempt to include activities that have these three components and utilize them in a variety of ways. The activities can include direct activities in which the students are engaged with the original data or sources of information; involve authentic settings where they are gaining experience by either doing or observing; or discussing, writing, or reflecting on what they are learning or how they are learning it. In addition, active learning activities should also include indirect activities. In this case, students may be provided with secondary sources of information through textbooks, lectures, or other publications; or presented with case studies, role-playing scenarios, or narratives (videos, written, or oral). A third and more recent type of active learning activity is the use of instructional technology in which the students utilize online course information, Web-based material, video lectures, course discussion boards, and reflections by others in and outside of the course and write their own reflections to the activities and learning experiences.

Many different learning activities can be used in the classroom. The challenge is to choose learning activities that will engage the students with the course material, meet the learning goals for the course, and provide evidence from which to assess student learning.

Integrating the Component Parts

The final step in the initial phase of building component parts is to integrate the component parts. Here, you need to check to make sure that there are intentional and balanced connections between the situational factors, learning goals, feedback and assessment, and the teaching and learning activities. These components need to be consistent and work together. Fink (2003) suggests creating a worksheet that contains the learning goals for the course and matching each learning goal with the procedure for assessing the students' learning and the learning activity that will be used. Then examine the worksheet to determine whether the components are integrated and whether the important connections are being made between these components. Thoroughly integrating the component parts allows the instructor to have a plan in place that will provide students with the best opportunity to successfully meet the learning goals for the course and to clearly demonstrate that they have met the learning goals. Furthermore, it allows the instructor to assess the quality of the course design.

Intermediate Phase: Assembling the Components Into a Coherent Whole

Creating the Course Structure

After you have completed the steps for the initial phase of course design, the next step is to assemble the components into an engaging course for the students. To do this, Fink (2004) suggests dividing the semester into four to seven segments, with each segment linked to an essential concept, issue, and/or topic of the course. For example, the segments for a language development course might include (1) introduction of the language terms and models of development; (2) normal development of the form, content, and use of language; (3) analysis of a typically developing child; and (4) atypical development and individual differences. Each segment of the language development course builds on the previous segment and links essential components of the course together. After the segments have been determined, they need to be arranged in a logical sequence, so that each segment builds on the previous one(s). Within each segment, the instructor needs to start by introducing the topic and then utilize course assignments to create learning opportunities for the students to apply the concepts and ideas (Fink, 2003, 2004). For example, in segment (1) of the language development example given previously, the instructor may start by presenting the definitions and models to the class and then incorporate activities such as having the students develop their own models of language development or having the students have a "meeting of the minds" in which the students are assigned to be the author of a specific model of development and then participate in a debate with the other groups regarding why their model is the best model of language development. During segment (2), students are asked complete homework assignments that require them to divide words into bound and free morphemes, calculate the type token ratio, calculate the MLU, and determine the conversational acts for specific groups of utterances. Thus, segment (2) requires that students utilize information from the previous segment in order to be successful on this assignment. The next segment could require students to complete their major project in the course. Here, students have to collect, orthographically transcribe, and analyze a language sample of a typically developing preschool age child. Again, to successfully complete this segment, students must utilize concepts and ideas that were learned in the previous segments. The fourth and final segment for the language disorders course could include teaching the students about atypical development and individual differences in language development. Students then would be asked to compare the data from their language sample with the data of their fellow classmates. Similarities and differences in the data would be discussed by the class as a whole, which would allow students to examine individual differences in typically developing children.

At this point in the design or redesign of the course, all we have done is to identify the segments. Although the preceding example provides specific tasks and teaching strategies, those tasks and strategies will be determined as we progress through the next steps.

Selecting an Effective Teaching Strategy

Fink (2003) makes a distinction between a teaching technique and a teaching strategy. "A *teaching technique* is a specific teaching activity" (p. 130), such as lecturing, class discussion, lab work, small groups, essays, or case studies. On the other hand, "a *teaching strategy* . . . is *a particular combination of learning activities in a particular sequence*" (p. 130). Therefore, a strategy is planned in such a manner that the instructor organizes a set of learning activities that will engage the students in activities that build on each other and result in maximizing student learning. This requires that the instructor determines which activities are needed to provide the prerequisite knowledge or skills for later performance and that, as students progress through the activities, they are provided with opportunities to practice previous abilities and develop later ones. The sequence can, and usually does, involve both in-class and out-of-class learning activities.

Therefore, in the language development course, the students initially completed specific homework assignments that asked them to divide words into bound and free morphemes and to calculate the MLU and TTR. The next segment then had the students utilize those concepts on an actual language sample. From there, they applied and compared their results to examine individual differences in normal language development. Therefore, each activity built on knowledge and skills from the previous segment and provided a variety of tasks from which the students learned the information.

A variety of teaching strategies can be used within a course. Some examples of teaching strategies include team-based learning, problem-based learning (see Chapter 6 for a discussion of problem-based learning and other teaching strategies), and accelerated learning.

Creating the Overall Scheme of Learning Activities

The next step in the process of designing a course that incorporates the concepts of creating significant learning is to integrate the course structure and the teaching strategy into the overall course design (Fink, 2003, 2004). To do this, we need to both differentiate and integrate the learning activities. Differentiation requires that we vary the activities within and between the days and segments of the course and that concepts and/or topics progress from easier to more challenging or complex. In addition, the course concepts and topics also need to be integrated. This integration needs to occur within and between the segments of the course. Therefore, at this stage, we need to determine what activities should come first versus last and what activities will allow the student to move between the first and last activities. When the overall scheme for the learning activities is complete, it is time to move to the final phase of creating significant learning.

Final Phase: Four Tasks to Finish the Design

Put Together the Grading System

As you enter the final phase of designing the course, the first step is to determine a grading system that will be fair for all students and educationally valid. It is important to remember that not every activity needs to result in a graded item. Some activities can just be for the experience of developing a specific knowledge component and/or skill. For example, in the hypothetical language development course when students developed their model of language development, it was an in-class assignment that was ungraded. In this example, the students had to examine the various models and think about the strengths and weaknesses of the models. From there, the students chose the elements for their own model of language development. The activity developed an understanding of the models of language development and the components of the various models. It also required that students integrate the information and apply it to create their own model.

For the activities that will be graded, it is important to make sure that a variety of activities are available and that all of the learning goals are measured in some manner. Furthermore, the weight of each learning activity needs to be determined. This means that activities that are more important should represent a larger part of the student's grade than those that are less important. To do this, the first step is to determine the key components in the grading system, such as the exams, projects, homework assignments, and so on. From there, you can determine the weight of each component, with the most critical components being worth more. In some courses, it may be important for you as the instructor to determine the weight of each component; whereas in other courses, you may decide that it will be determined by the students in the class. Either way is fine, provided that a plan is in place to determine the weight of each component at the beginning of the term.

Identify What Might Go Wrong

With grading system in hand or to be determined by the students, the next step is to critically evaluate the course one more time to determine whether any problems exist with the course as it has been designed. The problems may be logistical problems, such as whether you have the clinical facilities to accommodate all of the students for an observational assignment. Or the problems may be that you have too many fantastic assignments that the students really will not have the time to complete all of them well. On the other hand, maybe you have not provided enough depth in one of the essential components, so the students may not be successful in later aspects of the course. Therefore, at this stage, it is time to step back and examine the course from a distance to make sure that it will work and that you have not missed any critical elements. However, remember that you will not be able to anticipate all of the possible things that could go wrong. If you have taught even just one course in your career, we are sure that, after teaching that course, you realized things that you could have or should have done differently. There always will be things to tweak and modify, but the goal of this stage is to try and catch the major and sometimes minor errors that occur as you design a course for the first time or redesign a course to create a significant learning environment.

Write the Syllabus

The course now is designed, and the potential problems have been identified and corrected. It is now time to write the syllabus for the students. Although syllabi vary greatly from one professor to the next and one institution to the next, some essential components need to be in all syllabi. First, the syllabus needs to contain identifying information about the professor, including name, e-mail address, phone number, office location, and office hours. It also needs to contain the course name, number, description, and learning goals, outcomes, or objectives, grading procedures, and course policies regarding attendance, submission of assignments, make-up exams, and academic honesty policy. The required textbook(s) and readings also need to be included on the syllabus. Finally, a list or discussion of the structure and sequence of the course activities needs to be included. This includes due dates for the major assignments and tests.

Evidence for Syllabus Construction. Many anecdotal articles are available that describe the purpose and/or elements to include when designing a course syllabus. For example, Albers (2003) discusses how a syllabus can be used as a teaching tool, evaluation tool, and as a tool for documenting scholarship. As a teaching tool, the syllabus can serve as a contract between students and instructor, a communication device, a plan, and as a cognitive map that creates the "thematic framework that assists students in organizing the component parts of the course into a conceptual whole" (Albers, 2003, p. 61). A second function of the syllabus is as a tool for evaluating teaching effectiveness. For many, if not all of us, we have been asked to include our syllabi in our promotion, tenure, or job applications. The syllabus has become a part of our teaching portfolios that is intended to provide evidence of teaching effectiveness (Albers, 2003). The third use of the syllabus is as a tool for documenting scholarship. The syllabus provides documentation that demonstrates an instructor's scholastic ability to "integrate isolated learning activities into a coherent meaningful whole" (Albers, 2003, p. 63). The syllabus can be assessed with regards to the scholarship of teaching by examining the curricular knowledge, subject matter knowledge, and pedagogical knowledge.

Parkes and Harris (2002) propose three purposes of a syllabus: a contract, a permanent record, and a learning tool. The purpose of a syllabus as a contract matches with aspects of Albers' (2003) concept of the syllabus as a teaching tool. Parkes and Harris's suggestion that a syllabus can serve as a permanent record overlaps with two aspects of Albers' concept of the syllabus as an evaluation of teaching effectiveness and as a document of scholarship. The one purpose that differs for Parkes and Harris is that the syllabus could be a learning tool. If a syllabus is well-designed, it will provide the students with information that assists them in being effective learners beyond the specific course for which the syllabus is designed (Parkes & Harris, 2002).

Many resources discuss syllabus design. For example, there is the learner-centered approach (O'Brien, Millis, & Cohen, 2008); integrating traditional and critical approaches (Flowerdew, 2005); universal design (Passman & Green, 2009); and the promising syllabus (Bain, 2004; Hirsch, 2010; Lang, 2006). The design approach that is chosen for the syllabus will determine the elements included and how they are presented. Since there are more than ample resources available regarding the items to include and avoid in a syllabus, we will instead provide you with recommendations as to what to consider when writing and presenting your syllabus to the class.

The syllabus typically serves as the first interaction between you and the students in your class. Therefore, it is important that your syllabus conveys the messages you intend to communicate. Most instructors want their syllabi to create a balance of being approachable and caring, yet rigorous, challenging, and task-oriented. Those first impressions can determine whether students feel they will be successful in a class or not and therefore, whether they stay in the class or drop it. Thompson (2007) observed 13 classrooms on the first day of class when the syllabus was presented, interviewed 19 teachers, and analyzed the instructor's syllabi to determine the communication strategies that were used when presenting the syllabus to students. Three recurring communication strategies—welcoming, tension balancing, and presentational—were identified as being used by the instructor to focus the student's attention. Welcoming strategies included getting acquainted, being positive and encouraging, selling the course, and using inclusive language. Instructors also use tension balancing strategies when presenting their syllabus to the class. These can include softening the blow by addressing fears about the course, providing rules about the course, negotiating power through the syllabus by presenting students with choices, and by using stories or questions to engage the students. The final strategy that Thompson noted was the use of presentational strategies, such as highlighting and elaborating or focusing attention through the use of classroom technology.

Now that the syllabus has been presented, how do students perceive it? Saville, Zinn, Brown, and Marchuk (2010) examined students' perceptions of teacher effectiveness when presented with a detailed versus brief course syllabi. Ninety-seven undergraduate psychology students participated in the study, with approximately half of the students receiving a brief (two-page) course syllabus and the other half receiving a detailed (six-page) course syllabus. The same general information was contained on both syllabi, but the detailed syllabus contained more information for each item. The students reviewed the syllabus and then were asked to complete a survey regarding the content of the syllabus, and a Teacher Behavior Checklist for the professor of the class. The study found no significant difference between the groups with regard to the questions about the syllabus content. However, significant differences were found on several measures. Students who viewed the detailed syllabus were significantly more likely to recommend the course to another student, take another course with the instructor, and rated the hypothetical instructor as possessing the qualities of a master teacher—approachable, caring, flexible, more prepared, cognizant of current information, and promoting critical thinking (Saville et al., 2010). The students who viewed the brief syllabus found the hypothetical instructor to be less caring about them. Saville and colleagues (2010) concluded that the more detailed syllabus may motivate students and foster positive attitudes, which may create a positive classroom atmosphere from which the instructor may have a greater impact on the students.

Garavalia, Hummel, Wiley, and Huitt (1999) examined 242 undergraduate students and 74 faculty members' perceptions of the important syllabi components. Both the faculty members and the students preferred a more comprehensive syllabus and felt that the syllabus should be flexible or able to be revised as the semester progressed. The students perceived the following components to be important for a syllabus: "basic format of the exams, length and format of required papers and projects, statement of course withdrawal policy, listing of day-to-day class activities, and specific goals/objectives for each topic" (Garavalia et al., 1999, pp. 14–16). Some of these findings are consistent with Becker and Calhoon (1999) who examined what information students attend to in a courses syllabus. In their study, 863 students rated attending to the dates of exams and assignments the highest or most important information that they attend to, while course information, withdrawal dates, and readings were rated the lowest. Significant differences were found between first-semester students and nontraditional students as to what information they attended to the most. The first-semester students attended to information related to the location of materials, support services, and policies on late assignments and academic honesty and attended less to information regarding tests and assignments. On the other hand, the nontraditional students attended more to the course goals, titles and authors of the readings, and type of assignment; the information regarding holidays, late assignments, and academic honesty policies were attended to the least. Knowing what students perceive as important on a syllabus, enables us to make sure we meet their perceived needs and help them to focus their attention on aspects that we, as instructors, feel are more important.

So, is there a way to structure our syllabi to obtain a more positive response to the syllabus? Yes, there is. Research has examined the use of positive and negative words in a syllabus and its effect on student assessment of the course (Ishiyama & Hartlaub, 2002). Eighty-eight students enrolled in political sciences courses were randomly assigned to one of two groups: use of punishing language on a course syllabus and use of rewarding language on the syllabus. The students were presented with a sample syllabus from an introductory political science course and then took a survey that asked questions about the instructor of the course based on the syllabus and demographic information regarding the student. Ishiyama and Hartlaub found significant differences between the groups. The students in the negatively worded (punishing language) group were more likely to state that they were uncomfortable in approaching the faculty member. In addition, the wording had more of an impact on first- and second-year students than on third- and fourth-year students. However, no significant difference existed between the groups for their ratings of how difficult the course would be, nor the likelihood that they would take the course based on the wording of the syllabus. Finally, it was found that when grade point average (GPA) was controlled for significant differences were found between the groups. The students in the punishing language group, who had GPAs of 3.0 or above, were more likely to view faculty members as unapproachable and the class to be more difficult. Furthermore, there were no significant differences between the groups for students with GPAs below 3.0. Therefore, students with higher GPAs were more sensitive to the language used on the syllabus.

Calhoon and Becker (2008) examined how frequently students used the course syllabus. To do so, 112 general psychology students were randomly assigned to one of three groups. The students completed a survey twice, once during either week 3, 5, or 7 and then again 6 weeks later. During the first survey, all of the students reported that still had their syllabus and 92.9% of the students had their syllabus in a binder or notebook. At the second survey, all of the students who participated reported that they still had their syllabi, and only one student did not know where it was. Furthermore, almost 60% of the students transfer information from the syllabus to a calendar or planner; with 95.5% transferring test dates, 84.1% transferring assignments, and 50% transferring reading assignments. During the second administration of the survey, fewer students reported checking their syllabus within the past week. The majority of the students stated that they consult the syllabus for homework assignments, a quiz in the next class, and topics to be covered in the next class. Furthermore, for courses with more homework assignments, students reported that they relied more heavily on the syllabus. Calhoon and Becker noted that the use of the syllabus was dependent on the content of the syllabus (e.g., more assignments, more detail about assignments). Students also reported that they used their syllabi more frequently earlier in the semester compared to later in the semester. One final point to mention is that, although students tend to transfer due dates to their calendar or planner, they still referred back to the syllabus for the due dates (Calhoon & Becker, 2008).

In summary, as you write that course syllabus, remember that the syllabus is your chance to set the tone for the course and make your first impression. The syllabus needs to be written with your students in mind. Are they traditional or nontraditional students? Upperclassman versus underclassman? What's their typical GPA? In addition to the knowing your students, you also need to make sure that your syllabus is written utilizing positive language and provides enough detail. When you think you have your syllabus in the form that you want, there is one more step. It is imperative that you reread the syllabus through the eyes of your students, making sure that the syllabus clearly and concisely conveys the information to your students. State the obvious, eliminate surprises, and format the document so that the most important information is easy to locate (Fisch & Dorow, 2010).

Plan an Evaluation of the Course and Your Teaching

The final step in creating significant learning is to design a plan that would evaluate the course and your teaching of that course to determine how the course is going and how the course went (Fink, 2003). This step provides you with the opportunity to gather multiple sources of information, such as self-evaluation, student evaluation, and/or other professors' evaluation regarding your teaching and course design. Some ways for you to self-evaluate include video or audio recording the course and critically evaluating what you are doing in the classroom setting. Students could be asked to write minute papers with regard to your teaching and/or how the course is going, things that are working for them, and things that are not. Students also could be asked to complete a survey regarding specific aspects of a course. Another source of information is to have another professor observe your class or interview the students in the class to examine how the class is going or how the class went. If you would like feedback on specific aspects of the course, it may be helpful to ask specific questions of the students or other professionals regarding those aspects of the course. For example, if you incorporated a new teaching strategy and you would like to know the students perspective, then the students could be surveyed regarding the strategy and its perceived usefulness in meeting the course learning goals.

When the plan is in place for how you will evaluate the course, then it needs to be implemented, and the information needs to be analyzed. This analysis will provide you with information as to which aspects of the course design were successful and which may need to be tweaked or discarded in the future. The goal is that this evaluation will lead to an even better teaching and learning experience for all involved.

Evidence for Creating Significant Learning

Both qualitative and quantitative research is available that supports the use of Fink's concepts of integrated course design as a method for creating significant learning in our classrooms. The research evaluates the use of the integrated course design in courses from a variety of disciplines including civil engineering (Kolar, Sabatini, & Muraleetharan, 2009), Spanish (Davis, 2009), economics (Miners & Nantz, 2009), musical forms and analysis (Kelley, 2009), philosophy and art history (Rose & Torosyan, 2009), virology (Mester, 2009), a hybrid course in education (Fayne, 2009), special education (Fallahi, Levine, Nicoll-Senft, Tessier, Watson, & Wood, 2009; Levine, Fallahi, Nicoll-Senft, Tessier, Watson, & Wood, 2008; Nicoll-Senft, 2009), federal income tax (Huber, 2009), e-commerce education in information technology (Tabor, 2005), biology (Fallahi et al., 2009; Levin et al., 2008; Tessier, 2007), biomolecular sciences: anatomy and physiology (Fallahi et al., 2009; Levin et al., 2008), lifespan human development course in psychology (Fallahi, 2008; Fallahi et al., 2009; Fallahi & LaMonaca, 2009; Levin et al., 2008), and the psychology of early childhood (Fallahi et al., 2009; Levin et al., 2008).

The qualitative studies have found that utilizing Fink's (2003) integrated course design has an impact on both the students and the faculty member. From an affective or emotional aspect, changes were noted in that there was an increase in student buy-in and ownership of the course (Miners & Nantz, 2009). It also was noted that students were more enthusiastic about the course (Davis, 2009). Changes were also discussed with regard to changes within the classroom environment, in which students were found to be more actively engaged within the course (Kolar et al., 2009; Mester, 2009; Miners & Nantz, 2009; Rose & Torosyan, 2009). This active engagement was demonstrated by students as they were learning from each other, sharing their work, and synthesizing information as a whole (Rose & Torosyan, 2009).

Although it is nice to find changes and affect changes within the classroom interaction, the main goal of course design is to increase student learning and knowledge. Changes in student knowledge and learning were consistently noted by the published studies. Specifically, it was found that students moved "far beyond foundational knowledge" (Kelley, 2009, p. 41) and were able to solve real-world problems (Huber, 2009). The students demonstrated enhanced performance, greater depth of knowledge, were highly creative, and were able to connect knowledge obtained in the course to other courses (Mester, 2009). In addition, students who participated in courses that utilized Fink's (2003) integrated course design to create significant learning were more reflective (Mester, 2009) and demonstrated greater depth in their thinking (Kelley, 2009). The students "learned different ways to synthesize the material, which helped in their learning how to learn" (Rose & Torosyan, 2009, p. 68). Finally, utilizing integrated course design developed students who were lifelong learners (Mester, 2009).

The impact of utilizing Fink's approach to course design has not only been on the students within the classrooms, but also on the faculty members incorporating this design. Faculty members made many positive comments. Huber (2009), for example, stated that she had found the "joy in teaching" and that her "passion for teaching has been invigorated" (p. 15); Kolar and colleagues (2009) stated that "teaching is more fun" (p. 94). Not only did the faculty members feel better about teaching, they grew professionally (Fayne, 2009) and found that creating significant learning enhanced their own scholarship (Mester, 2009). As their scholarship was enhanced by this process, the faculty members also learned that they would need "to refine our course designs not once, but continually, to improve both student engagement and our own" (Rose & Torosyan, 2009, p. 68). Across the board, from one study to the next, the faculty members were realistic in the work involved in making the change to an integrated course design, while at the same time they found it to be a positive and rewarding teaching and learning process.

In addition to the qualitative evidence available in support of the Fink's creating significant learning, quantitative studies also support the use of this design. The first of the studies to be published was by Tessier (2007), in which he compared a traditional lecture-style approach to small-group peer teaching (SGPT) approach for teaching preservice teachers about basic biology concepts. The goal of the study was to determine whether the approach to teaching the course material (i.e., lecture vs. SGPT) affected the students' foundational knowledge of biology. Although Tessier's study did not incorporate all of the aspects of Fink's taxonomy, it does provide initial insights into the idea of creating significant learning. Specifically, Tessier (2007) found that students performed significantly better on content taught by each other on the SGPT days than material presented through lecture. Therefore, when students are engaged in active learning tasks, they demonstrated improved learning of foundational knowledge.

A group of faculty members at Central Connecticut State University, along with some other colleagues, have published several studies (Fallahi, 2008; Fallahi et al., 2009; Fallahi & LaMonica, 2009; Levine et al., 2008; Nicoll-Senft, 2009) regarding the results they achieved after designing or redesigning their courses utilizing Fink's concepts. These faculty members designed courses for five undergraduate courses and one graduate level course across four disciplines. Within each course, students were administered pre- and postsemester assessments, and data were analyzed within and between courses (Levine et al., 2009). Fallahi and colleagues (2009) reported the statistical results of the study and found significant improvements across all four disciplines in foundational knowledge, application, the human dimension, and learning how to learn. Improvements were also found in the dimensions of integration and caring; however, these changes were not found to be significantly different. For the caring dimension, the results could have been due to the ceiling effects of the measure, as there was limited potential for growth in this score when the pretest score was near the ceiling (Fallahi et al., 2009). Similar results were found in another study by Fallahi (2008), when she compared traditionally lecture-based course design to a redesigned course that was designed and taught based on Fink's model of creating significant learning. Students in the redesigned course performed significantly better on measures of foundational knowledge, application, and the human dimension. Furthermore, students in the redesigned course demonstrated improvements in their performance on integration, but no significant changes or trends were noted in performance on items related to learning how to learn or caring. In summary, the course redesigned based on Fink's creating significant learning was better than the traditional lecture-based course on teaching foundational knowledge, application, integration, and the human dimension (Fallahi et al., 2009).

In summary, both the qualitative and quantitative evidence lends support for the use of Fink's taxonomy for creating significant learning. Although the process initially is time consuming, it has lead to improved learning by students and a renewed passion for teaching by the faculty members incorporating it into their courses.

Application of Fink's Creating Significant Learning

Based on the overview of Fink's (2003) recommendations for creating significant learning, Vignette 4–2 and Vignette 4–3 will provide you with some example applications of Fink's approach.

Vignette 4–2. Application of Fink's Concepts for Creating Significant Learning: Language Development

General Type of Significant Learning	Course Goals— Students will be able to . . .	Assessment	Activity
Foundational knowledge	Describe models of language acquisition. Describe approaches for analyzing syntax, phonology, morphology, semantics, and pragmatic abilities.	Exam 1 Participation in class discussions	Create your own model of language development (in-class activity) Homework activities on creating list of analysis approaches.
Application	Apply course knowledge to language sample examples of a typically developing child.	Graded homework assignments Participation in classroom discussions Exam 2	Utilize Retherford's CD on assignments • MLU • Scavenger hunts — syntax and phonology • NP and VP Elaboration • TTR
Integration	Apply classroom concepts to analyze the morphological, syntactic, semantic, and/ or pragmatic characteristics of the language sample that the student collected. Discuss and interpret the results.	Exam 1 & 2 Homework assignment grades Participation in class discussions PBL rubric grades	• Language Sample PBL part 1 (language transcription and MLU) and part 2 (analysis and interpretation)

continues

Vignette 4–2. *continued*

General Type of Significant Learning	Course Goals— Students will be able to . . .	Assessment	Activity
Human dimension	Become aware of how environmental, cultural, cognitive, and social aspects influence language development	Participation in classroom discussions	Dear Abby Assignment on own reading development
Caring	Become aware of the complexity of language development	In-class assignment on language sample results	Class discussion comparing language sample results
Learning how to learn	Reflect on their own learning.	Written reflection on their own learning process and appraisal of their abilities to analyze a language sample	Reflection of PBL assignments

Vignette 4–3. Application of Fink's Concepts for Creating Significant Learning: Research Methods in Communication Disorders

General Type of Significant Learning	Course Goals— Students will be able to . . .	Assessment	Activity
Foundational knowledge	Levels of Evidence Based Practice (EBP) Demonstrate an understanding of the . . . • methodological aspects of qualitative and quantitative research	On-line quiz on EBP Grading of APA chapter summaries and questions	EBP presentation Linguisystems EBP APA chapter summaries and questions

Vignette 4–3. *continued*

General Type of Significant Learning	Course Goals— Students will be able to ...	Assessment	Activity
Foundational knowledge *continued*	Demonstrate an understanding of the ... • ethical treatment of participants. • APA publication rules.		
Application	Critically evaluate published research articles and determine level(s) of evidence.	Rubric grade on PBL #1	PBL#1 Individual and group critique of assigned peer-reviewed article
Integration	Design an appropriate and doable case study EBP research project for a patient in the Speech Clinic.	Rubic grade on PBL#2 final research proposal	PBL #2 Research proposal
Human dimension	Become more confident in their ability to critique and design clinical research.	Pre- and post-survey on research Written reflection on process	PBL #1; PBL #2; and Class discussions
Caring	Demonstrate an appreciation of research methodology and their ability to do research.	Pre- and post-survey on use of research	Class discussions
Learning how to learn	Reflect on their own learning and provide recommendations for future classes.	Written reflection on process Class discussion on process and recommendations for future classes	Letter to next year's research methods class

Concluding Remarks

Now that you have planned your design or redesign of the course, you need to consider several other details. As mentioned, Chapters 6 and 7 will be important chapters to consult as you design your course. Chapter 6 provides you with ways to engage the student in learning, whereas Chapter 7 provides you with a variety of ways to assess student learning. However, prior to providing those details, it is important to consider the most effective ways to communicate course information to your students, and the next chapter does that.

References

Albers, C. (2003). Using the syllabus to document the scholarship of teaching. *Teaching sociology, 31*(1), 60–72. Retrieved from http://www.jstor.org/pss/3211425

American Speech-Language-Hearing Association. (2009a). *Knowledge and skills acquisition (KASA) summary form for certification in Speech-Language Pathology.* Retrieved from http://www.asha.org/uploadedFiles/certification/KASASummaryFormSLP.pdf#search=%22KASA%22

American Speech-Language-Hearing Association. (2009b). *Knowledge and skills acquisition (KASA) summary form for certification in Audiology.* Retrieved from http://www.asha.org/uploadedFiles/certification/KASASummaryFormAud.pdf#search=%22KASA%22

Bain, K. (2004). *What the best college teachers do.* Cambridge, MA: Harvard University Press.

Becker, A. H., & Calhoon, S. K. (1999). What introductory psychology students attend to on a course syllabus. *Teaching of Psychology, 26*(1), 6–11.

Bloom, B., & Krathwohl, D. (1956). *Taxonomy of educational objectives: The classification of educational goals.* New York, NY: Longmans, Green, Co.

Calhoon, S., & Becker, A. (2008). How students use the course syllabus. *International Journal for the Scholarship of Teaching and Learning, 2*(1), 1–12. Retrieved from http://www.georgiasouthern.edu/ijsotl

Childre, A., Sands, J. R., & Pope, S. T. (2009). Backward design. *TEACHING Exceptional Children, 41*(5), 6–14.

Davis, D. D. (2009). Bringing language to life in second-year Spanish. *New Directions for Teaching and Learning, 119,* 17–23. doi: 10.1002/tl360

Fallahi, C. R. (2008). Redesigning a life span development course using Fink's taxonomy. *Teaching of Psychology, 35,* 169–175. doi: 10.1080/00986280802289906

Fallahi, C. R., & LaMonaca, F. H. (2009). Creating significant learning experiences in a large undergraduate psychology class: A pilot study. *Journal of Excellence in College Teaching, 20*(1), 87–100.

Fallahi, C. R., Levine, L. E., Nicoll-Senft, J. M., Tessier, J. T., Watson, C. L., & Wood, R. M. (2009). Using Fink's integrated course design: How a book changed our students' learning, our university, and ourselves. *New Directions for Teaching and Learning, 119,* 43–52. doi: 10.1002/tl363

Fayne, H. R. (2009). Using integrated course design to build student communities of practice in a hybrid course. *New Directions for Teaching and Learning, 119,* 53–59. doi: 10.1002/tl364

Fink, L. D. (2003). *Creating significant learning experiences: An integrated approach to designing college courses.* San Francisco, CA: Jossey-Bass.

Fink, L. D. (2004). *Designing courses that help students learn: A self-directed guide to designing courses for significant learning.* Workshop presented at the University of Virginia. Retrieved from http://trc.virginia.edu/Workshops/2004/Designing_Courses_2004.htm

Fisch, L. A., & Dorow, L. G. (2010). Syllabus redesign: Strategies that support students with disabilities. *The Teaching Professor, 24*(8), 4.

Flowerdew, L. (2005). Integrating traditional and critical approaches to syllabus design: The "what," the "how," and the "why?" *Journal of English for Academic Purposes, 4,* 135–147. doi: 10.1016/j.jeap.2004.09.001

Garavalia, L. S., Hummel, J. H., Wiley, L. P., & Huitt, W. G. (1999). Constructing the course syllabus: Faculty and student perceptions of important syllabus components. *Journal of Excellence in College Teaching, 10*(1), 5–12.

Hirsch, C. C. (2010). The promising syllabus enacted: One teacher's experience. *Communication Teacher, 24*(2), 78–90. doi: 10.1080/17404621003680880

Huber, M. M. (2009). Shoeboxes and taxes: Integrated course design unleashes new creativity for a veteran teacher. *New Directions for Teaching and Learning, 119,* 9–15. doi: 10.1002/tl.359

Ishiyama, J. T., & Hartlaub, S. (2002). Does the wording of syllabi affect student course assessment in introductory Political Science classes? *PSOnline,* 567–570. Retrieved from http://www.apsanet.org

Kelley, B. C. (2009). Inspiration and intellect: Significant learning in musical forms and analysis. *New Directions for Teaching and Learning, 119,* 35–41. doi: 10.1002/tl.362

Kolar, R. L., Sabatini, D. A., & Muraleetharan, K. K. (2009). Sooner City: Reflections on a curriculum reform project. *New Directions for Teaching and Learning, 119,* 89–95. doi: 10.1002/tl.368

Lang, J. M. (2006). The promising syllabus. *Chronicle of Higher Education, 53*(2), 114. Retrieved from Academic Search Complete.

Levine, L. E., Fallahi, C. R., Nicoll-Senft, J. M., Tessier, J. T., Watson, C. L., & Wood, R. M. (2008). Creating significant learning experiences across disciplines. *College Teaching, 56*(4), 247–254.

Mester, J. C. (2009). Integrated design of a virology course develops lifelong learners. *New Directions for Teaching and Learning, 119,* 71–79. doi: 10.1002/tl.366

Miners, L., & Nantz, K. (2009). More significant and intentional learning in the economics classroom. *New Directions for Teaching and Learning, 119,* 25–33. doi: 10.1002/tl.361

Nicoll-Senft, J. M. (2009). An "extreme makeover" of a course in special education. *New Directions for Teaching and Learning, 119,* 81–87. doi: 10.1002/tl367

O'Brien, J. G., Millis, B. J., & Cohen, M. W. (2008). *The course syllabus: A learner-centered approach* (2nd ed.). San Francisco, CA: Jossey-Bass.

Parkes, J., & Harris, M. B. (2002). The purposes of the syllabus. *College Teaching, 50*(2), 55–61. Retrieved from EBSCO Publishing.

Passman, T., & Green, R. (2009). Start with the syllabus: Universal design from the top. *Journal of Access Services, 6,* 48–58. doi: 10.1080/15367960802247916

Rose, M., & Torosyan, R. (2009). Integrating big questions with real-world applications: Gradual redesign in philosophy and art history. *New Directions for Teaching and Learning, 119,* 61–70. doi: 10.1002/tl.365

Savillle, B. K., Zinn, T. E., Brown, A. R., & Marchuk, K. A. (2010). Syllabus detail and students' perceptions of teacher effectiveness. *Teaching of Psychology, 37,* 186–189. doi: 10.1080./00986283.2010.488523

Tabor, S. W. (2005). Achieving significant learning in e-commerce education through small business consulting projects. *Journal of Information Systems Education, 16*(1), 19–26.

Tessier, J. (2007, January/February). Small-group peer teaching in an introductory biology classroom. *Journal of College Science Teaching,* 64–69.

Thompson, B. (2007). The syllabus as a communication document: Constructing and presenting the syllabus. *Communication Education, 56*(1), 54–71. doi: 10.1080/03634520601011575

Wiggins, G., & McTighe, J. (1998). *Understanding by design* (1st ed.). Alexandria, VA: Association for Supervision & Curriculum Development.

Wiggins, G., & McTighe, J. (2005). *Understanding by design* (Exp. 2nd ed.). Alexandria, VA: Association for Supervision & Curriculum Development [electronic version]. Retrieved from http://www.site.ebrary.com lib/bwc/Doc?id=10081770&ppg=25

Wiggins, G., & McTighe, J. (2007). *Schooling by design: Mission, action, and achievement.* Alexandria, VA: Association for Supervision & Curriculum Development.

5

Communication in the Classroom

> *There is a difference between knowing and teaching and that difference is communication in the classroom.*
> —Hurt, Scott, & McCroskey, 1978, p. 3

When we first came across this literature, our first thought was that it must be very similar to the literature about communication with which we are familiar from our own discipline. We are not only knowledgeable about communication literature, we are proficient communicators. We are particularly effective communicating with our clients and their families, and we have spent hours communicating effectively, in just the right way, about evaluation results, prognoses, and treatment outcomes.

We have learned, however, that research has shown that communication with students in the classroom is unique and bears consideration. A number of important reasons exist to give serious thought to classroom communication. In this chapter, we look at how communication skills impact teaching and learning. We explore constructs specific to how teachers communicate with students and how to improve communication in online learning, thereby improving student outcomes. Numerous studies have demonstrated that an instructor's communication style in the classroom influences students' cognitive learning, how they feel about the subject, and how they behave as a learner in that classroom.

Communication routinely is considered an essential aspect of effective teaching. Studies of mastery teaching consistently indicate that expert teachers have excellent communication skills in the classroom (Garmston, 1994; Hativa, Barak, & Simhi, 1999; Rubin & Feezel, 1986; Rubin & Morreale, 1996). Being an effective communicator consistently and historically is considered a competency needed to be an effective teacher (Polk, 2006; Smith, 1980. In seminal research of teacher communication styles, Norton noted "Teacher effectiveness is shown to be intrinsically related to the way one communicates" (Norton, 1977, p. 526).

Instructional Communication Competence

Teacher communication skills, often referred to as instructional communication competence in the communication sciences literature, can be highly influential regarding students' perceptions of the instructor, the course, and their own learning outcomes (Gorham & Christophel, 1992; Kerssen-Griep, 2001; Worley, Titsworth, Worley, & Cornett-DeVito, 2007). Instructional communication competence has been defined (Worley et al.) as:

> The teacher-instructor's motivation, knowledge, and skill to select, enact, and evaluate effective and appropriate verbal and nonverbal, interpersonal and instructional messages filtered by student-learners' perceptions, resulting in cognitive, affective, and behavioral student-learner development and reciprocal feedback. (p. 208)

Recent research has worked to whittle this lengthy definition down to identify key elements of communication behaviors that faculty would benefit from incorporating into their classrooms. This definition also focuses attention on the value of the teacher-learner interaction, critical to the success of EBE, as described in Chapter 2.

In studies of the types of communication behaviors students either prefer or expect, being learner-centered and engaging or enthusiastic appear high on the list (Gorham & Christophel, 1992; Houser, 2004, Worley et al., 2007). It is noted that learner-centered communication, as described in Chapter 3, is particularly critical to students we often label "nontraditional" because they are older than 23 years of age. Attention to the preferences of these students is particularly important as the shift for enrollment at most universities indicates that the nontraditional student represents 43% of the student population (Houser, 2004). In a study of teacher communication acts that increase student motivation, Kerssen-Griep (2001) identified communication activities that students indicated were important. Students reported that they valued when teachers communicate that students share ownership of the class, such as when teachers refer to "our" class and provide opportunities for input regarding the course. When teachers convey respect for individual students through inclusive language, it creates an environment that facilitates students voicing their opinions and taking risks sharing their thoughts. Respect through courteous listening, engaging in dialogue, using students' names, and openness to student input, must be conveyed in order for the learning environment to be perceived as safe by learners. Students want instructors to demonstrate interest in their efforts and contributions to the class, through either verbal or written feedback. Students reported appreciating communication that encourages them to attempt higher-order learning, such as that requiring application, analysis, and synthesis, and that inspires confidence in their ability to be successful in these tasks. Finally, teacher communication that validates the students' efforts and encourages them to keep improving was important to the students. Many of the items on this list reflect that students value communication behaviors that support them and make them feel valued as learners in the classroom (Kerssen-Griep, 2001).

In an effort to learn more about how to improve instructional communication competence, a study examined the views and behaviors of teachers who had demonstrated communication mastery in their teaching based on receipt of a national teaching award (Worley et al., 2007). In this qualitative study, faculty participants were interviewed and observed teaching. Inductive analysis of the data revealed remarkable consistency and similarities across the teachers in their communication behaviors and reflections on communication. One lesson, that was of particular interest to us as speech-language pathologists and audiologists, was that the teachers noted that not only do they rely on the feedback from their students to guide their communication, but also to determine how a class was progressing based on how much time the students spent talking during class, such that if the teacher is doing less talking than the students, she perceives that she is doing a better job teaching. The master teachers indicated that it is critical to be adaptable with your communication style so that you can match your style or approach to the context of your classroom. Study participants highlighted the value of interpersonal relationships, on a professional level, which should be developed through communication inside and outside of the classroom. These efforts help to validate the students as individuals and accept their roles within the learning environment. This last recommendation did not include that teachers be inappropriately friendly or develop relationships with students beyond the boundaries of the professional role. However, the teachers felt that it is necessary to recognize that we are engaged in interpersonal relationships with our students and that our communication should facilitate the development of interpersonal affinity between students and teachers. Engaging in "rapport-talk" (Worley et al., 2007, p. 230) before and after class, such as asking how their weekend was, or discussing a popular novel you are reading, helps the students feel comfortable with the teachers and encourages them to feel that they can approach the teacher readily.

Immediacy and Clarity

Immediacy

To further understand the value of teachers' perceived approachability, we must explore the literature regarding the relationship between classroom communication and student learning by exploring two instructional communication frameworks that our colleagues in communication science have studied extensively. The first important framework is *immediacy,* which refers to teacher communication characteristics that influence the perception of psychological and physical closeness between teacher and student (Frymier, 1994; Frymier & Weser, 2001; Moore, Masterson, Christophel, & Shea, 1996, Nixon, Vickerman, & Maynard, 2010). Immediacy behaviors are those that influence the students' perceptions that we, as faculty, are approachable and accessible. For example, you might think of immediacy, loosely translated, as the students' sense that were they to have concerns about class, they could come to you and talk about them. The research regarding immediacy is vast and extensive, reaching back to the early 1970s when Mehrabian first introduced the concept (Nixon et al., 2010). Mehrabian's first explanation as to why teacher immediacy was important was through the approach-avoidance theory which suggests that "people approach what they like and avoid what they don't like" (Nixon, Vickerman, & Maynard, 2010, p. 492), In other words, when teachers make themselves likeable or approachable, students are less likely to avoid interactions with them.

As research into immediacy evolved from the initial description, it was separated into two distinct categories that are still discussed today: verbal immediacy and nonverbal immediacy, although there is some contention regarding the role of each in the classroom, which we will explore later in this chapter. Verbal immediacy is the set of language based behaviors that create a sense of connection between us and our students, and nonverbal immediacy refers to the set of nonverbal behaviors, such as tone of voice, that contribute to that sense of connection for our students. In 1988, Gorham first introduced a scale that she used in her research to have students assess their teacher's immediacy. Not all items in her scale may be socially acceptable in today's society by the diverse population of students that we have in our classrooms. More recent research has investigated the variety of responses students from different cultures to immediacy behaviors; however, most items in the original scale are still relevant for many of us and are worth considering. In recent years, researchers have questioned the relative value of verbal immediacy relative to nonverbal immediacy; however, there continues to be evidence that both types are valuable for the classroom. Verbal and nonverbal behaviors associated with immediacy are summarized in Table 5–1. When a teacher is said to rate well on the scale, she is said to have high immediacy, and when ratings are poor, she is said to have low immediacy.

Over the years, this list has been modified by a variety of researchers for a number of research purposes. As a research tool, it has provided us with a greater understanding of the significance and value of teacher immediacy. As a feedback mechanism, it can

Table 5–1. Immediacy Behaviors

Verbal Immediacy Behaviors
Items associated with increased immediacy • Uses personal examples or shares experiences she/he has had outside of class. • Asks questions or encourages students to talk. • Participates in discussions based on a topic a student brings up even when this is not part of his or her lecture plan. • Uses humor in class. • Addresses students by name. • Addresses me by name. • Initiates conversations with individual students before, after, or outside of class. • Has initiated conversations with me before, after, or outside of class. • Refers to class as "our" class or what "we" are doing. • Provides feedback on my individual work through comments on papers, oral discussions, etc. • Asks for students' opinions about an assignment, due date, or discussion topic. • Invites students to telephone or meet with him/her outside of class if they have questions or want to discuss something. • Asks questions that solicit viewpoints or opinions. • Praises students' work, actions, or comments. • Willing to discuss things unrelated to class with individual students or with the class as a whole. • Is addressed by his/her first name by the students. **Items associated with decreased immediacy** • Refers to class as "my" class or what "I" am doing. • Calls on students to answer questions even if they have not indicated that they want to talk. • Asks questions that have specific, correct answers. • Criticizes or points out faults in students' work, actions, or comments.

Table 5–1. *continued*

Nonverbal Immediacy Behaviors
Items associated with increased immediacy • Gestures while talking to the class. • Makes eye contact with the class while talking. • Smiles at the class as a whole, not just individual students. • Touches students in class. • Moves around the classroom while teaching. • Has a very relaxed body position while talking to the class. • Smiles at individual students in class. • Uses a variety of vocal expressions while talking to the class. **Items associated with decreased immediacy** • Sits behind desk while teaching. • Uses monotone/dull voice when talking to the class. • Has a very tense body position while talking to the class. • Sits on a desk or in a chair while teaching. • Looks at the board or notes while talking to the class. • Stands behind podium or desk while teaching.

Source: Based on Gorham, J. (1988). The relationship between verbal teacher immediacy behaviors and student learning. *Communication Education*, 37.

provide faculty with informal, low-stakes information regarding how your students perceive you as a communicator in the classroom. If you choose to use it in your classroom, it can be adapted in ways that are appropriate for your teaching style and context. For example, if you teach in an institution that frowns on the use of professors' first names by students, or you are not comfortable with that, that item can be deleted from your questionnaire.

In recent years, the measure of verbal immediacy has come under attack as being an invalid measure (Richmond, McCroskey, & Johnson, 2003). Rather than view verbal immediacy as a set of behaviors that create an approachable, accessible teacher, as Mehrabian did, Richmond and colleagues described "the principle of immediate communication" indicating that "the more communicators employ immediate behaviors, the more others will like, evaluate highly, and prefer such communicators; and the less communicators employ immediate behaviors, the more others will dislike, evaluate negatively, and reject such communicators" (Richmond, McCroskey, & Johnson, p. 505). Their belief was that the verbal immediacy scale was simply a measure of verbal behaviors that effective teachers employ, rather than isolating immediacy-related behaviors. They, therefore, encouraged us, saying that it is "better to think of immediacy simply as a nonverbal construct" (p. 506). However, Wilson and Locker's (2007) data suggests that measures of teacher effectiveness only "moderately overlap" with the item from the verbal immediacy scale and that the earlier criticism is unfounded. They suggest instead that "an effective teacher might not be immediate, but an immediate teacher likely would be seen as effective by his/her students" (p. 8).

Although what verbal immediacy represents has been questioned, the value and role of nonverbal immediacy has been free of controversy. As researchers have become more convinced of the value of nonverbal immediacy, they have sought to expand the items that are valid and reliable. Richmond, McCroskey, & Johnson (2003) created two scales that can be used by the teacher to rate his or her own nonverbal immediacy and by his students to rate the teacher's nonverbal immediacy. Their research found the two new scales to be valid and reliable. The scales include the items on Gorham's original immediacy scale, Table 5–1, and add more specific items that address vocal expressiveness, such as variety and animation, eye contact, facial expressiveness, body language, gestures, and proxemics. The debate regarding the value of verbal immediacy is shared with you here for several reasons. First, should you find yourself intrigued by this construct and decide to incorporate it into your own SOTL research, you should be aware of the dispute as you delve into it further. Clearly, there are arguments and data for both views. The second reason for sharing this information is to help you take the value of immediacy into perspective. We are not suggesting that all good teachers are immediate and therefore that teachers with poor immediacy cannot be effective. However, we have found the behaviors that are included in the original immediacy behavior scale to be valuable for guiding faculty in improving their classroom communication and their ability to help the students feel more connected to them. Whether immediacy is truly a separate construct from teaching effectiveness or not, it is clear that students have more favorable responses to teachers with high immediacy.

No matter which view you take on verbal immediacy, there can be little doubt from the wide-ranging research that has been completed in the last 20 years that teacher immediacy has a powerful impact on the students. Here, we will explore the relationship between immediacy and a variety of student outcomes. Early research (Gorham, 1988) identified strong positive correlations between both verbal and nonverbal immediacy and affective learning as well as student perceptions of cognitive learning. Later studies have suggested that nonverbal immediacy has a higher correlation to cognitive and affective learning (Christensen & Menzel, 1998; Comstock, Rowell, & Waite, 1995; Witt & Wheeless, 2001). It has been suggested that one possible reason for increased learning in the presence of immediacy is that students feel more positive affect for the instructor and for the subject when the teacher increases the feelings of approachability verbally and nonverbally (Christensen & Menzel, 1998; Rodriguez, Plax, & Kearney, 1996). It also has been posited that teacher immediacy results in increased student attention and will "stimulate arousal" (Houser & Frymier, 2009, p. 39). The combination of stimulation and attention, along with positive feelings toward the instructor that results from immediacy may in turn result in improved cognitive learning (Rodriguez, Plax, & Kearney, 1996). Allen, Witt, and Wheeless (2006) conducted a rigorous study of the relationship between teacher communication behaviors and instructional outcomes for students and found that in addition to the positive affect for the course and the instructor, noted previously, students reported greater motivation with an immediate teacher. These results have been supported by researchers who have examined the relationship between affective learning and motivation, suggesting that both increased affective learning and motivation in the presence of teacher immediacy are likely to lead to improved student success (Pogue & AhYun, 2006). Students of teachers with immediacy also use more direct communication strategies with their teacher to request assistance or clarification while students of low-immediacy teachers are likely to turn to other sources of information for support or assistance (Myers & Knox, 2001). Additionally, Vignette 5–1 illustrates how you can begin establishing your immediacy on the first day or your course.

> **Vignette 5–1.** Teacher Immediacy on the First Day of Class
>
> On the first day of class, I am sure to be there early. By being there before them, I have a few minutes to ensure that the classroom is set up the way I prefer it, which is typically in either small group clusters or in a circle, whichever can be managed in the room. Placing students in these arrangements, rather than in straight rows facing me, tells them right away that, just because I am the teacher, I am not going to be the sole focus of their classroom interactions and learning. As they are able to see each other easily, they will be able to communicate with each other more readily. This sets the tone for the class being "ours," not "mine."
>
> Before the students arrive, I also write a very brief, skeletal outline in the upper right corner of the white board. This outline is typically only about five to seven items long and each item might be only a word or two. For example, in the first day of diagnostic methods class, the outline might read
>
> - Syllabus Review
> - Introductions
>   - You
>   - Me
> - Learning Goals
> - Begin Screening vs. Evaluation
> - Next Week
>
> This outline does a few things for our class. As students arrive in the class for the first time, it lets them know that they always have a place to look to see what the plan for the day is (and I tell them this, too). It gives them a sense of what to expect for the day, which decreases learner anxiety by increasing their ability to anticipate accurately. It tells them that, during the introductions, I want to learn about them, and they will get to learn about me. It also tells them that we will cover what to expect for the term, which is foremost on their minds. Finally, it lets them know that, yes, indeed, they actually will be learning something on the first day of our class.
>
> After letting them know about the outline and the fact that they can count on it to be there every week, we review the syllabus because

Vignette 5–1. *continued*

I think that this is what students are most anxious to learn on that first day. They want to know what the work load will be, what form it will take, and understand what will be expected of them. By getting this out of the way first, I can hold their attention for the rest of the time with less distraction and apprehension. Next, we move on to introductions. I begin by asking them to tell me their first names, and then I ask them to share something that will tell me a little about who they are. To be honest, I do this to cover my own inadequacy of a faulty memory for names. I remember other details well, though; having them share something helps me associate their names with their faces. This also adds to their understanding that I care about who they are as individuals. As students go around the room sharing whatever piece of information that I have asked for, usually other students interject small comments, and there is some banter back and forth that I participate in. For a class of 20 students, this only takes about 5 minutes and is well worth the time to give them the cue that I want to hear their voices in class. Through this exercise, I have learned that I have a woman hockey player in my class, a student who tried sky diving during her break, and that I share some musical tastes with some students. All of these things help us connect on an interpersonal level, as well as helping me remember their names.

Before we move onto talk about the serious stuff, I move on to introducing myself. Only I don't really introduce myself. I share with them that I have learned over the years that whatever I can tell them about myself may not be what they actually want to know. So, rather than tell them things that they may not care about, I give them the opportunity to ask me what they want to know either about me as a teacher, as an individual, or about the class. I ask them to get together into groups of two to three students and accomplish two tasks. First, I ask them to exchange e-mail addresses or phone numbers so that, in the event that they miss class due to illness, they have someone whom they can contact to ask questions or get notes. This creates a sense of a community, or social presence, for the people who may have come to class not knowing anyone. Their second task is that, as a group, they need to create a couple of questions that they want to ask me. I let them know that they can ask me about personal or professional issues and that I reserve the right to not answer, although I have

continues

Vignette 5–1. *continued*

> never actually had to invoke that right. Students work together, again an early step in creating social presence for them, and develop their questions. By doing this in a group, no one has to take ownership of questions that they might be embarrassed about asking either. I then give them time to ask their questions aloud so that the whole class hears. Over the years, I have been asked about my research agenda, my clinical interests, my own musical interests, where I have travelled to, where I went to school, and one of my favorite questions, "What pushes your buttons most that students do?" After the students have asked their questions, we move on to the next item on the list.
>
> I learned the technique of allowing students to ask me questions instead of telling them what I want them to know from a colleague, Dr. David Coffey at Grand Valley State University, who referred to it as a "Piece of Me" exercise that he had learned many years earlier at a workshop. I pick and choose how to answer the questions. I don't get too personal, but I do use any question I can as an opportunity to share small things about myself that I think will make the students more comfortable in the learning environment. Answering their questions lets them know that I am open to questions in general and that I am a person that they can connect with, and it gives them the information that they really do want to know about me. Through this exercise, and all of the other communication efforts I have made in our first 20 minutes together, I have started to establish my immediacy quickly for the students and set the tone that I hope will foster a positive learning environment for the rest of the term.
>
> Examples of items you can ask the students to share with you on the first day of class:
>
> 1. Tell us the most fun thing you did on your vacation.
> 2. Share with us something you did for the first time ever this past year.
> 3. Tell us something that would surprise us to know about you.
> 4. What was the last music concert you attended?
> 5. What is your favorite food?
> 6. What is your favorite television show or movie?
> 7. What is the best gift you ever gave or received?

Clarity

The second instructional framework that has been studied in college teaching is *clarity*. Clarity is when "an instructor is able to effectively stimulate the desired meaning of course content and processes in the minds of students through the use of appropriately structured verbal and nonverbal messages" (Chesebro & McCroskey, 1998, p. 262). This definition of clarity is fairly broad; however, Sidelinger and McCroskey (1997) note that it often includes the ability to explain information effectively through elaboration on concepts, structuring tasks, and scaffolding content. Additional behaviors that increase teacher clarity include soliciting questions from students, use of examples, and use of clear, concise language, particularly with new material (Chesebro & McCroskey, 2001; Myers & Knox, 2001). In an effort to create a brief measure of clarity for use by students in the college classroom, Chesebro and McCroskey (1998) created the Teacher Clarity Short Inventory (TCSI), which they determined in their study to be both reliable and valid. The inventory is reproduced in Table 5–2. Teacher clarity has been correlated highly with immediacy, particularly nonverbal immediacy (Sidelinger, & McCroskey, 1997).

Past studies have demonstrated that when students have teachers with good clarity, they experience a variety of positive learning outcomes similar to those experienced by students of immediate teachers (Houser & Frymier, 2009) In a number of studies, clarity was highly correlated with student affective learning (Sidelinger & McCroskey, 1997), and with cognitive learning (Chesebro & McCroskey, 2001; Hativa, 1998; Titsworth, 2001). A number of explanations exist as to why clarity improves student learning. It may increase cognitive learning because clarity facilitates note taking by students (Titsworth, 2001). It may increase affective learning because when teachers demonstrate clarity, students are more likely to have positive affect for the instructor, for the course, and to be more motivated due to students' decreased apprehension levels (Chesebro & McCroskey, 2001). Further, it has been noted that students feel more positively toward a teacher whom they feel is credible and capable of teaching them effectively. When students perceive instructors to have clarity, they are more likely to use overt-information seeking strategies with teachers, just as they do when the teachers have

Table 5-2. Teacher Clarity Short Inventory

> **Strongly Agree = 5, Agree = 4, Undecided = 3, Disagree = 2, Strongly Disagree = 1**
>
> 1. My teacher clearly defines major concepts (explicitly states definitions, corrects partial or incorrect student responses, refines terms to make definitions more clear).
> 2. *My teacher's answers to students' questions are unclear.
> 3. In general, I understand my teacher.
> 4. *Projects assigned for the class have unclear guidelines.
> 5. My teacher's objectives for this course are clear.
> 6. My teacher is straightforward in her or his lecture.
> 7. *My teacher is not clear when defining guidelines for out-of-class assignments.
> 8. My teacher uses clear and relevant examples. (He or she uses interesting, challenging examples that clearly illustrate the point. He or she refines unclear student examples. He or she does not accept incorrect student examples.)
> 9. *In general, I would say that my teacher's classroom communication is unclear.
> 10. My teacher is explicit in her or his instruction.

*Items should be reverse coded.

Source: From Chesebro & McCroskey (1998). The development of the teacher clarity short inventory (TCSI) to measure clear teaching in the classroom. *Communication Research Reports, 15*(3), p. 264. Copyright © 1998 by James McCroskey. Reprinted with permission.

immediacy, rather than relying on observations and third-party information gathering strategies (Myers & Knox, 2001). Finally, clarity has been shown to have a strong positive correlation with students' satisfaction and, thus, instructor and course evaluations (Hativa, 1998; Sidelinger, & McCroskey, 1997).

It should be noted that significant similarities exist between the positive outcomes associated with teacher clarity and immediacy. Improved learning, ratings of instructors, and motivation all have been associated with these two instructional communication constructs. The combination of immediacy and clarity was highlighted in a recent study when the influence of teacher communication behaviors on students' sense of learner empowerment was examined (Houser & Frymier, 2009). In this study, empowerment referred to the learners' feelings of motivation to perform tasks, that the tasks are perceived to be meaningful, that they as students will be competent to complete the tasks, and that their efforts can have an impact on the environment. Based on the teachers' characteristics of clarity and immediacy, the authors were able to predict the students' feeling of empowerment within the classroom context, thus affirming that teacher communication behaviors can have a strong influence on the student learning experience.

Teacher Transparency

Communication science research also has shed light on the relationship between students' perceptions that their teacher cares about them and their learning outcomes. Immediacy data suggests that if students feel that the teacher is connected with them through immediacy, then they are likely to have positive affect for the teacher and perform better in the class. It may be that the immediacy helps to promote "perceived caring" (Teven & McCroskey, 1997, p. 1). Teacher behaviors that convey concern regarding their well-being, such as demonstrating empathy, understanding, and responsiveness will be viewed as caring by their students. When teachers are perceived to be caring by their students, students are more likely to evaluate the instructors and the courses more favorably. In addition, they report that they learn more in the course, both cognitively and affectively (Teven & McCroskey, 1997). Additionally, teachers who have high immediacy are perceived to be more caring than teachers who have low immediacy (Teven, 2001).

The intersection between caring and immediacy is interesting because measures of caring are based on relational perceptions, whereas measures of immediacy are based on behaviors (Teven, 2001). In an effort to uncover what teachers with immediacy and clarity do to convey that they are caring, Ginsberg (2007a, 2007b) examined the information communicated by these teachers to their students. The results indicate that teachers who are clear and immediate share information that suggests to the students that they care about them, that they are humanistic in nature, and how they view the teaching and learning process. The content of the communication that lets students see who their teacher is, creating *teacher transparency* (Ginsberg, 2007a, 2007b). Faculty who have teacher transparency consistently were found to be immediate, clear, humanistic, and caring.

Additionally, consistent with the literature regarding immediacy and perceived caring, students of teachers with transparency reported being more motivated to achieve for the teacher and in that class. Students often cited their understanding of the transparent teacher's educational philosophy in explaining why they were motivated to work hard to be successful. The students not only felt that they understood their teacher's view of learning and good teaching, they often were able to explain it in very similar terms to how the teachers with transparency did (Ginsberg, 2007a, 2007b). In contrast, students of teachers who did not have transparency noted their lack of insight as to why they were being asked to do particular tasks by a teacher as a reason that they were not enthused about the class and associated assignments. This resistance to teachers with limited transparency is consistent to the passive resistance students demonstrate with teachers who have low immediacy, which the low transparency teachers also had (Burroughs, 2007). Teachers' philosophies of education are the "filter" (Hativa, 1998, p. 355) through which their actions in the classroom and with students pass. Students understanding the nature of this filter may help them feel empowered to find the learning activities more meaningful and valuable (Houser & Frymier, 2009).

Self-disclosures are one of the key mechanisms that provide students with the information about their teacher, including that they are caring (Ginsberg, 2007a, 2007b, 2007c). Self-disclosures that are used honestly were an element that contributed to positive ratings by students (Scott & Nussbaum, 1981). Although self-disclosures are known to be one of the characteristics that influence student perceptions of immediacy, Ginsberg's study analyzed the content of the self-disclosures. Faculty self-disclosures typically are part of the professor's dialogue with the students and are embedded in the context of the classroom discussions. Self-disclosures that are professional in nature include comments regarding previous professional experiences, such as "I treated people with this condition when I worked at the University Hospital," or "In the 25 years that I have been evaluating hearing, I have only had that problem with a client once." From these small references to the instructor's clinical experiences, for example, the students decide that the instructor has increased credibility because he or she has experienced a clinical situation first hand or because the teacher has a large number of years of clinical experience. In clinical fields, these professional-experience self-disclosures also may further convince the students of the value of the information being shared.

Faculty professional self-disclosures in this study also addressed the teacher's philosophy of teaching and learning. These can be particularly critical for motivating students to be successful in your classroom. Teachers with transparency routinely shared information with students relevant to their expectations regarding learning and their philosophy of teaching (Ginsberg, 2007a, 2007b). When interviewed about their teachers, students of transparent teachers typically were able to indicate what their teacher's expectations were for their own learning outcomes. They noted their teacher's philosophy about teaching and connected it with their willingness to work hard because they understood the purpose or value of the effort. Students of teachers who were not transparent were less motivated by academic challenges as they noted that they were unclear about what the expectation or purpose of the assignment was. Understanding teachers' beliefs helps students understand the purpose of tasks or expectations that are imposed on them, which further motivates them to be successful (Ginsberg, 2007a; 2007b; Hativa, 1998).

Although professional self-disclosures tend to help the students value the information being taught and improve the teacher's perceived credibility, personal self-disclosures can increase the students feeling of knowing who the teacher is as a person and thus connecting with them. Many colleagues would point out that we do not want our students to know many personal things and we would agree. The study did not advocate that personal self-disclosures should compromise teachers' privacy or would make anyone uncomfortable. You may feel comfortable disclosing many small, benign pieces of information to your students. When a teacher mentions her daughter, who is in college nearby, during the course of talking with students about stress, it tells the students that the teacher understands the student experience from multiple perspectives. A teacher commenting to the class that he found some useful information for his students while visiting a friend at the hospital indicates he is thinking about the course outside of the classroom. These comments share with the students the kind of person the teacher is, conveys to them that he is thinking about their course outside of the classroom, and models for the students making connections between the outside world and what is being learned at school.

Social Presence

Over the past 10 years, the body of literature regarding communication for teaching and learning with technology has grown exponentially as the prevalence of online and blended or hybrid formats, which include face-to-face and online learning combined, have increased dramatically (Garrison, Cleveland-Innes, & Fung, 2010). Many theories have been put forward to account for the role of communication, particularly between teacher and student, in the online environment. One of the constructs related to the early work in immediacy, particularly in online learning settings, is social presence. Social presence was a concept first described to refer to a variety of contexts and refers to the way in which a communication medium influences the degree of intimacy experienced by individuals. As education became more computer based, such as in distance learning, the idea of social presence became relevant to learning and student success online. Researchers began describing social presence as the sense of belonging to a community that is developed by teachers and is experienced by students in online learning environments (Gunawardena, 1995, Gunarwardena, & Zittle, 1997). The definition was expanded in 2010 to "the ability of participants to identify with the community (e.g., course of study), communicate purposefully in a trusting environment, and develop inter-personal relationships by way of projecting their individual personalities" (Garrison, Cleveland-Innes, & Fung, p. 32).

It has been hypothesized that when students feel they are part of a learning community, even when they cannot see one another, that they will be more likely to persist in their educational endeavors and to be more satisfied with their learning experiences (Rovai, 2002). This has been born out in the research. Just as immediacy has been found to be valuable in the traditional classroom, the value of social presence to the students has been extensively demonstrated in online education. Garrison and colleagues (2010) noted in their study of causal relationships in the online learning context that social presence is a mediating factor in student success as it allows students to develop trusting relationships online and work collaboratively, which improves the context for learning. Instructor communication to students through e-mails in the online course context enhanced student motivation as well as the attitudes of the students toward the course and the instructor (Legg & Wilson, 2009). Social presence, fostered through course design that includes social interaction online, such as through collaborative learning, can reduce the feelings of student isolation (McInnerney & Roberts, 2004). Social isolation not only negatively may influence the students' view of learning and perceptions of the learning experience, but may result in poor retention for a class or program.

Increasing Social Presence

Social presence often is described in terms of immediacy as many instructors use immediacy in this setting to create the social presence between themselves and their students. The significant challenge is, of course, how to achieve immediacy and social presence in a medium that typically does not provide for visual cues and face-to-face interaction. Woods and Ebersole (2003) developed a list of strategies that are useful in developing a sense of community in online environments that they refer to as "Community Building Activities (CBAs)" (p. 3). The first CBA that is recommended is to create a space in the online learning platform for students to share a sense of themselves with the rest of the class. This sets the stage for the members of the class, even though they don't know what they look like, to make associations with the student as an individual, for example, identifying interests, hobbies, or goals. This also can be accomplished through an "introductions" exercise in which students and the professor share a little about themselves early in the semester.

This increases immediacy and a sense of who is in the community. McInnerny and Roberts (2004) refer to this introductory process as a "forming stage" or a "warm up period" (p. 78). They note that it also can be used to make introductions about how to use and navigate the online learning platform. Giving students an opportunity to figure out how the system works is also important for decreasing the anxiety associated with learning and being graded using unfamiliar software (Ginsberg, 2008).

Many of the behaviors or tasks that Woods and Ebersole (2003) recommend are designed to increase immediacy indirectly; however, they also suggest several activities that are specifically intended to improve immediacy. Two key mechanisms are responding in a timely manner and the use of emoticons in electronic communications. In terms of timing, it has been suggested that faculty respond to threaded discussions or e-mails within 24 hours (Woods & Ebersole, 2003). Lack of timely electronic communication from instructors in online learning settings has been found to be a source of frustration and negative views of learning for students (Ginsberg, 2008). Using emoticons (the small images of a smiling face or keystroke combinations that signify emotion, such as ;-) for a smiling, winking face) are suggested as CBAs that will improve nonverbal immediacy. In essence, the emoticons can signify humor, similar to tone of voice or facial expression, and have been found to reduce the perception of anger (Woods & Ebersole, 2003). Additionally, the authors suggest that e-mail communication should be personalized on occasion to create the sense of connectedness with students. This might take the form of asking how a student is feeling if they have e-mailed you that they have been ill, or giving encouragement, such as noting that they made a nice contribution to the threaded discussion that day. These e-mails need not be long, but they appear to play a critical role in creating that sense of being connected to the teacher and that the teacher is someone who cares. Personal e-mails are also valuable when a class meets in person as well. Legg and Wilson (2009) found that when teachers sent a brief, positive welcome e-mail to a class one week before the first day of class, it improved significantly the students' motivation and attitude toward the teacher as well as their perception of the course for the duration of the term.

Additional activities that are likely to increase social presence for the students include the use of audio or video materials in your course platform, which are discussed in Chapter 6. This may be as complex as creating a short video of you demonstrating a clinical activity, such as creating a hearing aid mold. A simple way to add audio to an online course is to take a PowerPoint presentation that you may have created to outline a specific lesson and narrate it with an audio-recording. Occasionally using either audio or video tapes allows students to see your face, hear your voice, and develop a sense of who you are as a person. Creating a personal space for the students to communicate privately, away from the instructors eyes, is another CBA that can be implemented on some platforms. These spaces can be labeled as chit-chat rooms or study rooms. The students are told that the instructor will not have access to them unless invited to do so. This creates opportunities for students to talk with each other, much in the same way as they do entering the classroom or during a brief break in a long class.

The use of synchronous communications, or communication that takes place at the same time, is recommended as a way to improve social presence (McInnerney & Roberts, 2004; Woods & Ebersole, 2003). Often referred to as live chats or chat rooms, this type of communication reduces perceptions of difficulties in communicating and feel more instantaneous. The student feels that he has greater access to the instructor and often the instructor is able to use more spontaneous, informal communication. Students who experience anxiety associated with not being able to get questions answered or clarification provided to them in a timely manner are likely to be appreciative of synchronous communication as well (Ginsberg, 2008).

Another mechanism for informal communication that is starting to be explored is the use of social networking for supplementing communication in online learning (Joyce & Brown, 2009). Social networking software, which may be referred to as Web 2.0, is software that allows members of the sites to create the content that others view and also to control who views it. Current popular examples include LinkedIn (http://www.linkedin.com) and Facebook (http://www.facebook.com). One of the benefits of the use of this software is that in addition to being free, the majority of our students already have accounts. With a reported 94% of college students having a Facebook account, it is safe to assume that they know how to use it, and therefore, will have less anxiety associated with it because it can be used for low-stakes purposes in the class (Ginsberg, 2008; Joyce

& Brown, 2009). The use of social networking must be associated clearly with learning and as an educational tool, which means that the instructor must be prepared to model and guide the students in its appropriate use. Opportunities for informal interaction around course content may lead to reducing the sense of isolation that can be associated with online learning. It is recommended for use in making introductions, allowing students to interact with each other, and for sharing resources that they find valuable (Joyce & Brown, 2009). It may be preferable for faculty to create a second work-related Facebook account to separate your personal communication from the communication with students that, while informal, is still professional. Overall comfort with using social networking and other informal electronic communication will vary from teacher to teacher and should be done in accordance with what seems appropriate for your relationship with your students and with what you are comfortable. For ideas on how to develop social presence and immediacy in your online or hybrid class, see Vignette 5–2.

This section would not be complete without a final note about the etiquette of communication in online courses. Just as we are responsible for creating safe, personally inviting and engaging atmospheres for learning in the classroom, we also are responsible for monitoring for behavior that threatens that sense of comfort and community online. Faculty using computers for learning, whether in a fully online course or a blended format, should be sure to review proper electronic etiquette, or netiquette. Fortunately, a number of Web pages are designed to teach people about netiquette, including Purdue University's OWL resource (http://www.owl.english.purdue.edu/owl/resource/636/01/) and the Albion page (http://www.albion.com/netiquette/). It may be beneficial to have a policy or a statement regarding adhering to the rules of etiquette that appears early in the course. One common problem in electronic communications that teachers need to be watchful for is "flaming" or posting of inflammatory, antagonistic messages, and e-mails. We need to let students know that this style of communication is not acceptable and that it will not serve them well as they move forward into the CSD professions either. Sharing netiquette information and making it explicit will help students feel more safe and secure in this learning environment (McInnerny & Roberts, 2004).

> **Vignette 5–2.** Developing Immediacy and Social Presence in a Hybrid Class

In a hybrid, or blended, format class, the teacher and students meet in a traditional face-to-face format for some portion of the semester and also use an electronic platform for part of the learning. In my dysphagia class, I wanted to be sure that the students understood a clear connection between both the content that they learned in each setting and also the learning communities that they are part of in both settings. I have learned from past experience that it is not safe to assume that students in a hybrid class automatically would experience the social presence of a classroom while in engaged in the electronic learning context. In fact, some students reported a distinct disconnect between the two settings, so I tried to design dysphagia to avoid that problem.

To make clear connections for the students between learning online and learning in the classroom, I set up the syllabus so that it would highlight these connections for them. The syllabus showed the students how the material that they read would be used to complete an online learning activity, which then would be the starting point for the in-class discussion the next time the class met. The syllabus thus increased continuity and clarity, as well as making clear my intentions in course design, which I hoped would increase my transparency, too. The syllabus also communicated to the students deadlines for all learning in all contexts so that there was little concern that information could not be organized all in one location. I provided the syllabus to the students in hard copy on the first day of class and posted it on the course home page as well.

In order to have the students feel engaged in true learning within a community online, I provided them with problem-based learning (PBL) activities each week (see Chapter 6 for a full discussion of PBL). Students were assigned to small groups, an average of four students per group, that were responsible for developing a feasible solution to a clinical problem. They needed to discuss the problem through the use of threaded discussions and create one final product as a result of that discussion, which would be turned in on behalf of the group. In short, the PBL that they received was a clinically realistic problem that they must solve as though they were each members of a small department working in a hospital. No specific responses or solutions expected, but

continues

Vignette 5–2. *continued*

rather the discussion and the final product had to reflect the content that had been learned, from readings, class discussions, and lecture material and had to be appropriate and feasible. An example of a clinical problem given the students was that they were charged with developing an intake form for a patient complaining of dysphagia that could be administered either verbally in a very brief period of time, or could be sent to the patient prior to the first visit.

To facilitate the use of threaded discussions online, the first assignment in the class was low stakes. They were told of the deadline for participation, but they also were told that, if they had any difficulty with technology, they could contact me to seek support with no penalty. They also were given access to the online course several days prior to the actual start date of the course. I provided them with the access information in a welcome e-mail. These opportunities to explore and ask for help without negative impact on their grades decreased their anxiety about relying on their ability to navigate course platform successfully. As threaded discussions began, I logged into each group's to make a small comment of encouragement to a few individuals or the group as a whole. This increased my online immediacy by being supportive, recognizing the value of students' efforts, and demonstrating that I was attending to the work that they were undertaking at the time. They knew that I was in each group with them and would on occasion address a question to me in this asynchronous setting. I also used individual e-mails to communicate words of encouragement or suggestions for their thinking based on the threaded discussions throughout the semester.

Although students in the small groups for the online setting were all in the same class together, they were not given time in the face-to-face class to meet and work. They were, however, expected to report out as a group when they returned to class after completing an online assignment. Each in-class meeting began with discussion about the outcomes of the online learning that had taken place prior to it. Although the students did not sit with their online groups, they were asked to share their insights, discussions, and results with the whole class, thus giving them another opportunity to strengthen their sense of being in a learning community. Giving the groups opportunities to report out to the class as a whole also reinforced the collaborative learning by bringing small group learning back to the larger class (see Chapter 6 for more discussion on collaborative learning).

Vignette 5–2. *continued*

> Finally, in a slightly modified version of using social networking software for online learning, I took advantage of the many dysphagia-related videos that have been posted on YouTube (http://www.youtube.com/). Fortunately, dysphagia lends itself well to videotapes. I created my own video channel, where I collected examples of quality videofluoroscopies and endoscopies that I felt were good enough for the students to learn from in the context of our class. I also found numerous educational videos that already had been posted by other academic programs, including by faculty at medical schools. I shared this "channel" with the students in class and showed them where the link in the online course was that would take them directly to the channel with one click. They were able to comment on what they saw there and were encouraged to identify video clips that they thought would make good additions to the channel. This was not an assignment for points; however, students appreciated the free access to videos in a format that they felt comfortable with and they were soon finding suggestions of quality materials that could illustrate what we had discussed in class or that they found useful to view. As the collection grew, credit was given to the student who found the item, further increasing both their sense of immediacy and social presence. Further, their ability to contribute to class content and teaching materials had the potential to empower them within the dysphagia course.

References

Albion (2006). *Netiquette home page*. Retrieved from http://www.albion.com/netiquette/

Allen, M., Witt, P. L., Wheeless, L. R. (2006). The role of teacher immediacy as a motivational factor in student learning: Using meta-analysis to test a causal model. *Communication Education, 55*(1), 21–31.

Burroughs, N. F. (2007). A reinvestigation of the relationship of teacher nonverbal immediacy and student compliance-resistance with learning. *Communication Education, 56*(4), 453–475.

Chesebro, J. L., & McCroskey, J. C. (1998). The development of the teacher clarity short inventory (TCSI) to measure clear teaching in the classroom. *Communication Research Reports, 15*(3), 262–266.

Chesebro, J. L., & McCroskey, J. C. (2001). The relationship of teacher clarity and immediacy with student state receiver apprehension, affect and cognitive learning. *Communication, Education, 50*, 1, 59–68.

Christensen, L. J., & Menzel, K. E. (1998). The linear relationship between student reports of teacher immediacy behaviors and perceptions of state motivation, and cognitive, affective, and behavioral learning. *Communication Education, 47*(1), 82–90.

Comstock, J., Rowell, E. B., & Waite, J. (1995). Food for thought: Teacher nonverbal immediacy, student learning, and curvilinearity. *Communication Education, 44*(3), 251–266.

Frymier, A. B. (1994). A model of immediacy in the classroom. *Communication Quarterly, 42*, 2, 133–144

Frymier, A. B., & Weser, B. (2001). The role of student predispositions on student expectations for instructor communication behavior. *Communication Education, 50* (4), 314–326.

Garmston, R. J. (1994). The listening presenter. *Journal of Staff Development 15*(3), 61–62.

Garrison, D. R., Cleveland-Innes, M., & Fung, T. S. (2010). Exploring causal relationships among teaching, cognitive, and social presence: Student perceptions of the community of inquiry framework. *Internet and Higher Education, 13*, 31–36.

Ginsberg, S. M. (2007a). Shared characteristics of college faculty who are effective communicators. *The Journal of Effective Teaching, 7*(2), 3–20.

Ginsberg, S. M. (2007b). Teacher transparency: What students can see from faculty communication. *Journal of Cognitive Affective Learning, 4*(1), 13–24.

Ginsberg, S. M. (2007c). Faculty self-disclosures in the college classroom. *The Teaching Professor, 21*(4), 5.

Ginsberg, S. (2008). Student anticipations and reactions to hybrid format education. *Perspectives Issues in Higher Education*, 76–82.

Gorham, J. (1988). The relationship between verbal teacher immediacy behaviors and student learning. *Communication Education, 37*, 41–53.

Gorham, J., & Christophel, D. M. (1992). Students' perceptions of teacher behaviors as motivating and demotivating factors in college classes. *Communication Quarterly, 40*(3), 239–252.

Gunawardena, C. N. (1995). Social presence theory and implications for interaction and collaborative learning in computers. *International Journal of Education Telecommunication, 1*(2/3), 147–166.

Gunawardena, C. N., & Zittle, F. J. (1997). Social presence as a predictor of satisfaction within a computer-mediated conferencing environment. *The American Journal of Distance Education, 11*(3), 8–26.

Hativa , N., Barak R., & Simhi E. (1999). *Expert university teachers: Thinking, knowledge and practice regarding effective teaching behaviors.* Retrieved from ERIC database. (ED 430 961)

Hativa, N. (1998). Lack of clarity in university teaching: A case study. *Higher Education, 36*(3), 353–381.

Houser, M. L. (2004). Understanding instructional communication needs of nontraditional students. *Communication Teacher, 18*(3), 78–81.

Houser, M. L., & Frymier, A. B. (2009). The role of student characteristics and teacher behaviors in students' learner empowerment. *Communication Education, 58*(1), 35–53.

Hurt, T. J., Scott, M. D., & McCroskey, J. C. (1978). *Communication in the classroom.* Reading, MA: Addison-Wesley.

Joyce, K. M., & Brown, A. (2009). Enhancing social presence in online learning: Mediation strategies applied to social networking tools. *Online Journal of Distance Learning Administration, 12*(4). Retrieved from http://www.westga.edu/~distance/ojdla/winter124/joyce 124.html

Kerssen-Griep, J. (2001). Teacher communication activities relevant to student motivation: Classroom facework and instructional communication competence. *Communication Education, 50*(3), 256–273.

Legg, A. M., & Wilson, J. H. (2009). E-mail from professor enhances student motivation and attitudes. *Teaching of Psychology, 36*(3), 205–211.

McInnerny, J. M., & Roberts, T. S. (2004). Online learning: Social interaction and the creation of a sense of community. *Educational Technology and Society, 7*(3), 73–81. Retrieved from http://www.ifets.info/journals/7_3/8.pdf

Moore, A., Masterson, J. T., Christophel, D., & Shea, K. A. (1996). College teacher immediacy and student ratings of instruction. *Communication Education, 45*(1), 29–39.

Myers, S. A., & Knox, R. L. (2001). The relationship between college student information-seeking behaviors and perceived instructor verbal behaviors. *Communication Education, 50*(4), 343–356.

Nixon, S., Vickerman, P., & Maynard, C. (2010). Teacher immediacy: Reflections on a peer review of teaching scheme. *Journal of Further and Higher Education, 34*(4), 491–502.

Norton, R. (1977). Teacher effectiveness as a function of communicator style. In B. Ruben (Ed.), *Communication Yearbook 1* (pp. 525–542). New Brunswick, NJ: Transaction.

Pogue, L. L., & AhYun, K. (2006). The effect of teacher nonverbal immediacy and credibility on student motivation and affective learning. *Communication Education, 55*(3), 331–344.

Polk, J. A. (2006). Traits of effective teachers. *Arts Education Policy Review, 107*(4), 23–29.

Purdue Online Writing Lab. (2011). *Email Etiquette*. Retrieved from http://owl.english.purdue.edu/owl/resource/636/01/

Richmond, V. P., McCroskey, J. C., & Johnson, A. D. (2003). Development of the nonverbal immediacy scale (NIS): Measures of self- and other-perceived nonverbal immediacy. *Communication Quarterly, 51*(4), 504–517.

Rodriguez, J. I., Plax, T. G., & Kearney, P. (1996). Clarifying the relationship between teacher nonverbal immediacy and cognitive learning: Affective learning as the central causal mediator. *Communication Education, 45*(4), 293–305.

Rovai, A. (2002). Building a sense of community at a distance. *International Review of Research in Open and Distance Learning, 3*(1), Retrieved from http://www.irrodl.org/index.php/irrodl/article/view/79/153

Rubin, R. B., & Feezel, J. D. (1986). Elements of teacher communication competence. *Communication Education, 35*, 254–268.

Rubin, R. B., & Morreale, S. P. (1996). Setting expectations for speech communication and listening. *New Directions for Higher Education, 96*, 19–29.

Scott, M. D., & Nussbaum, J. F. (1981). Student perceptions of instructor communication behaviors and their relationship to student evaluation. *Communication Education, 30*, 44–53.

Sidelinger, R. J., & McCroskey, J. C. (1997). Communication correlates of teacher clarity in the college classroom. *Communication Research Reports, 14*(1), 1–10.

Smith, B. O. (1980). *A design for a school of pedagogy*. Washington, DC: U.S. Department of Education.

Teven, J. J. (2001). The relationship among teacher characteristics and perceived caring. *Communication Education, 50*(2), 159–169.

Teven, J. J., & McCroskey, J. C. (1997). The relationship of perceived teacher caring with student learning and teacher evaluation. *Communication Education, 46*(1), 1–9.

Titsworth, B. S. (2001). The effects of teacher immediacy, use of organizational lecture cues, and students' notetaking on cognitive learning. *Communication Education, 50*(4), 283–297.

Wilson, J. H., & Locker, L. (2007). Immediacy scale represents four factors: Nonverbal and verbal components predict student outcomes. *Journal of Classroom Interaction, 42*(2), 4–10.

Witt, P. L., & Wheeless, L. R. (2001). An experimental study of teachers' verbal and nonverbal immediacy and students' affective and cognitive learning. *Communication Education, 50*, 327–342.

Woods, R., & Ebersole, S. (2003). Becoming a "communal architect" in the online classroom-integrating cognitive and affective learning for maximum effect in web-based learning. *Online Journal of Distance Learning Administration, 6*(1). Retrieved from http://www.westga.edu/~distance/ojdla/spring61/woods61/html

Worley, D., Titsworth, S., Worley, D., & Cornett-DeVito, M. (2007). Instructional communication competence: Lessons learned from award-winning teachers. *Communication Studies, 58*(2), 207–222.

6

Engaging the Learner

> *The art of teaching is the art of assisting discovery.*
> —Mark van Doren

By and large, course instructors in undergraduate and graduate CSD programs are able to teach and research in areas of personal clinical and theoretical interest. Most faculty would consider this to be one of many "perks" of life in academia, as they are able to pursue an understanding of issues germane to specific topics within the practice of speech-language pathology and/or audiology. This pursuit of a discipline-specific specialization encourages faculty to become focused and engaged in learning more about the topics in which they're most interested. In turn, faculty can pass on their interests in various areas of specialization to their students within the classroom. In doing so, faculty share subjects they find to be interesting with students on a regular basis. But the question remains: Are faculty successful in making course topics as dynamic for students as they are for the faculty member in question? As faculty, many of us have had the experience in which despite being absolutely passionate about the topic we're covering in class on a given day, our students don't seem remotely excited to be part of the class at all. Why is this? What keeps the course instructor's enthusiasm from being contagious for students? We would argue that the issue here is engagement. While faculty are engaged with their topic, students aren't always feeling the connection between the course content, the faculty member, and their own interests. This has the potential to become a roadblock to learning, as we know from many different studies that students will learn more as they feel more engaged with the learning process centric to a given course.

Consistent with our discussion in Chapter 3, we are advocates for active involvement in learning in order to maximize student engagement and acquisition of new knowledge. To fully realize this ideal, faculty need to utilize teaching strategies and practices that complement the vibrancy of their course content. Techniques to help engage students as partners in their learning are simply complements to an overall learner-centered instructional focus. Our belief matches existent EBE outcomes: Students will be more motivated to learn course material and will retain it for longer if faculty can catch and hold the interest of their students. Fortunately, many evidence-based techniques can be applied to the design and implementation of a given course that have been proven to engage students as active partners in the learning process. A variety of these techniques are enumerated within this chapter.

Collaborative Learning Techniques

Collaborative Learning Techniques (CLTs) are useful to employ in order to provide balance to the structure of class meetings so that lecture isn't the only method being utilized to teach and learn. CLTs are strategies or ideas for structuring interactions within a class meeting or online learning environment wherein students are able to work together to drive and focus their learning with the facilitation and oversight of their course instructor.

Ideally, within the blueprint for each class meeting, faculty should try to ensure that interactions are set up to foster collaboration between course stakeholders in a number of ways: from teacher to students, from students to teacher, and from student to student. Some faculty might be reluctant to allow for a collaborative approach to teaching and might hesitate to let students assist in the construction of their own knowledge. Yet, realistically, audiology and speech-language pathology students are pursuing training in a very clinically oriented field of study, one that demands that practitioners work collaboratively with other specialists in various settings. We strongly feel that providing a learning experience that does not foster a sense of cooperation and collaboration is an absolute disservice for our students. Undoubtedly, students must have individual core knowledge as specialists. That said, we would argue that part of our duty as teachers is to also impart an appreciation for seeking the perspectives and expertise of others in a responsible, appropriate fashion. CLTs are useful in helping to facilitate that differentiated sort of class interaction and constitute a series of varied teaching methods that can be utilized during class meetings, as appropriate.

Encouraging High-Quality Class Discussions

Due in large part to faculty who realize that talking about ideas and communicating them to others has tremendous pedagogical value, class discussion has been and remains one of the most popular instructional methods used in higher education in the United States (Barkley, Cross, & Major, 2005). Research would support the use of class discussion as being an effective teaching strategy, as even three decades ago evidence existed to support class discussions as leading to use of higher level thinking skills (Smith, 1977).

Despite the regularity with which class discussions are used, it is widely thought that setting up successful discussions is not an easy task (Barkley, Cross, & Major, 2005). Many faculty have reported feeling as though students are uninterested in contributing to class discussions and have noticed the same students being contributors class after class with few novel voices heard as part of the discussion. Students themselves sometimes will prefer to be passive learners, seeking for knowledge to simply be imparted to them (Visconti, 2010). Others students might hesitate to contribute to a discussion due to anxiety that they might seem less intelligent than they would like to be viewed. Perhaps students feel that their perspective wouldn't be valued. Whatever the obstacle, and despite the widespread use of in-class discussions as central to many faculty members' teaching, issues do exist that keep the potential for high-quality class discussions from being fully realized.

The evidence base for using in-class discussions as a teaching tool is clear, though, despite roadblocks that might exist. McKeachie (1999) indicated that when compared to lecture-based learning, class discussions led to better retention of information and overall deeper understanding of course content. Good-quality class discussions lead to learning that is active in nature and encourages perspective-taking amongst students (Roehling, Vander Kooi, Dykema, Quisenberry, & Vandlen, 2011). Many agree that the key to establishing high-quality class discussions lies within how the groundwork is laid by faculty to encourage an environment conducive to sharing thoughts and ideas (Barkley, Cross, & Major, 2005; Ezzedeen, 2008; Roehling et al., 2011).

Establishing an Environment for Discussion

What is meant by establishing an environment conducive to class discussion? In large part, we refer to the need for faculty to adjust certain variables, which are well within their control to lay a purposeful foundation to encourage student engagement. In short, establishing an environment for discussion is considered to be anything course instructors do to set the stage for student engagement, lay out expectations for students, and devise questions likely to generate good class discussion. Wade (1994) found that the most common reason for students not engaging in class discussions was attributed to specific teacher practices. Thus, we would suggest a need to examine with a critical eye those practices we engage in as teachers, to ensure that we aren't mitigating our chances of effectively engaging students due to a practice that we can adapt or change easily. We must create a classroom climate for interaction amongst students and faculty.

Searching to identify factors associated with high levels of student participation in the college classroom, Rocca (2010) undertook an extensive literature review examining studies conducted over the last 50 years. Overall, Rocca's findings indicated that "creating a supportive climate has repeatedly been shown to increase participation and it is strongly recommended that professors work to create such an environment in a variety of ways" (p. 205). This study yielded several important, evidence-based suggestions for establishing an environment for class discussions. We have divided these suggestions into three major, recurring themes: demonstrating respect for students, providing support for students, and asking the right questions of students. These suggestions are summarized in Table 6–1 along with specific teacher practices, which fall into each theme, and a rationale that explains the importance of each area for the creation of positive classroom climate.

Table 6–1. Evidence-Based Teacher Practices for Establishing Positive Classroom Climate[1]

Behaviors Fostering Positive Class Environment	Specific Teacher Practices	Rationale for Practice
Demonstrating respect for students	• Faculty praise students' contributions to class discussions. • Faculty are perceived as valuing student input/ideas. • Faculty are able to call on specific students by name, even in large classes. • Faculty are patient, providing ample student response time (3–5 seconds). • Faculty use good interpersonal skills and eye contact to engage students in dialogue. • Faculty are inclusive of varied perspectives within a given discussion.	These practices are associated with higher levels of student comfort/confidence and have been proven to lead to increased participation in class.

continues

Table 6–1. *continued*

Behaviors Fostering Positive Class Environment	Specific Teacher Practices	Rationale for Practice
Providing support for students	• Faculty provide positive verbal feedback to encourage student contributions. • Faculty are "good listeners." • Faculty display enthusiasm for teaching and subject matter. • Faculty facilitate discussion effectively. • Faculty emphasize collaboration over competition. • Faculty set expectations that are clearly communicated to students and provide ample guidance through the learning process.	Students are more likely to ask questions and offer comments/ ideas in class discussions when they perceive a teacher as being supportive of their efforts.
Asking the right questions of students	• Faculty propose questions that encourage interpretation, rather than reporting of facts. • Faculty pose questions to which they don't necessarily know the answer. • Faculty self-disclose appropriate amounts of personal information to help students relate to faculty more effectively.	Faculty who engage in these practices are perceived as being reciprocal and respectful toward students and are considered to value interaction among teachers and students.

[1]Summarized from Rocca (2010).

We have several other considerations for faculty looking to adapt their practices to positively influence their classroom environment:

- Explicitly model your class discussion philosophy. If you want students to engage in intelligent conversation in the classroom setting you need to model that behavior in a professional, nonjudgmental, approachable manner (Roehling et al., 2011).
- Interact with students before and outside of class. Weaver and Qi (2005) suggest that this assists students in developing respectful, reciprocal relationships with faculty, which can increase student comfort levels with in-class participation.
- Know, accept, and accommodate for your situational constraints. Situational constraints are those aspects of your teaching that you have little control over: time of day a class is offered, class size, classroom resources, etc. You might not be able to change a large class into a smaller one, but you can work around this constraint by utilizing techniques proven to work with larger groups of students such as changing room arrangement to reflect a more conversational set up (Fritschner, 2000), engage in small group breakout discussion sessions (Davis, 1993), or using proximity to engage students throughout the room (Rocca, 2010).
- Allow for students to prepare thoughts and ideas prior to class meetings (particularly early in the semester when students are still getting used to your class). Small assignments can be assigned to allow for "the confidence that comes with advanced preparation" (Rocca, 2010, p. 206). These assignments can serve as the starting point for class discussions, rather than asking students to address questions with little preparation.

Techniques for Peer Teaching

Sometimes, the best teacher isn't a teacher at all. Rather, sometimes students learn best from interacting with peers, navigating new information and generating knowledge in a reciprocal, interactive manner. This phenomenon is referred to as peer teaching and occurs when students play a dual role (both teacher and student) in the pursuit of learning about a particular topic. As is the case with many pedagogical techniques in which students are active in their pursuit of learning, faculty members act as facilitators during peer teaching experiences, ready to support students as needed to best drive student learning.

Barkley, Cross, and Major (2005) describe peer teaching as an interdependent process wherein students "cooperate rather than compete, as each student has a stake in the successful learning of others" (p. 133). At its core, peer teaching is a collaborative process that requires students to actively engage in working with others to achieve a common goal, an endeavor ideal for future clinicians who will work in conjunction with peers in related professions everyday to diagnose and treat communication-based disorders. Christiansen and Jensen (2008) found that peer teaching specifically targets clinical skills, such as collaboration, reflection, and professional communication, which have the potential to drive higher-level affective learning, as described previously in Chapter 3. Beyond these affective skills, it has been reported that peer teaching has the potential to affect change in how students think about learning. Loke and Chow (2007) found that though peer teaching, students gain a sense of responsibility for learning and are taught about *how* to learn, in general.

So how does peer teaching actually work? Faculty create situations for students to work in small groups to share and discuss information relevant to the class in question. These collaborative discussions can be formal (structured as part of class time/class expectations) or informal (students work together outside of class meeting time). Students engage in various collaborative practices to encourage learning. Barkley, Cross, and Major (2005) describe a variety of CLTs, which set the stage for peer teaching. These are summarized briefly here:

- *Use note-taking pairs:* This CLT is meant to be used to help students collaborate to improve the quality of their class notes. Students pool their course notes together to form a more complete, comprehensive version of notes for a given topic. This can happen over the course of one class period or for longer, depending on teacher and student needs. This CLT could be used in an anatomy and physiology course in which students could use a course period prior to an exam to review and share their class notes, filling in missed information and asking questions

related to any course content they failed to understand in prior class meetings.
- *Establish a learning cell:* Students using this CLT craft questions about some course experience/topic (e.g., readings, lecture, discussion) and take turns testing one another with their derived questions. Students collaborate to master course content in an interactive, team-based fashion. This might be another CLT that could be applied as a pre-exam learning strategy. Students in any class could make up sample exam questions and test one another's knowledge. Some questions derived by students could even be incorporated into the "real" exam given by the course instructor.
- *Operate within a fishbowl:* For this CLT to be facilitated, two groups of students are formed: the inside of the circle and the outside of the circle. The inside of the circle group is given a topic to critically consider. They discuss and debate the topic, while the outside circle group critiques the content of the discussion from an outside perspective. This fishbowl CLT has the dual purpose of exposing students to practice with class discussion and providing opportunities for students to model and/or observe group interactions in a collaborative discussion-based setting. Thus, students in a cleft-palate course could discuss a particular case study, weighing the pros and cons of assessment and treatment approaches while classmates observe the process and note anything with which they strongly agree or disagree. A large class exchange could be held after the fishbowl experience to bring everyone back together and share ideas and solutions to any issues that were raised.
- *Organize role play:* Role play is considered a CLT because in the context of taking on a role that a student might never have played before, students have the opportunity to gain experiential knowledge though interaction with peers. Students have the opportunity to practice perspective-taking, expand their knowledge base, and apply theory to practice in a rudimentary manner. Students in a speech sound disorders course could set up a role play situation in which one student acted as a clinician and one acted the role of a child with the phonological process of stridency deletion. The student who acted as the clinician would gain experience with test administration, interpretation, and phonetic transcription, and the student who acted the role of the child

would have to develop a deep understanding of stridency deletion in order to produce an accurate portrayal of the phonological process in question.

- *Teach using jigsaws:* Jigsaws are designed by faculty, who want to engage in the training of relative experts on given course topics. Students are grouped twice to maximize learning: (1) Students are grouped to gain expertise on a given topic, investigating and studying the topic to fully understand it within the context of a class; then (2) break up into small, secondary groups in which the experts trained in the first groupings of students teach the rest of the class about their topic. Thus, with this CLT, students learn and share their learning in a collaborative manner. Students in a language disorders course might use jigsaws to learn about the etiologies of language disorders. Students can be split up into six groups to study various known causative/contributing factors for language impairment (e.g., mental impairment, specific language impairment, autism, hearing impairment). When each group finds the information required to explain the factor they've researched and discuss how their particular etiological factor could contribute to or cause language impairment, the class can be reconfigured into six different groups with one "expert" from each etiology group being in each new group. The experts can inform the others about their etiological condition, sharing information to form a complete picture of the different causes/contributing factors for language impairment.
- *Create test-taking teams:* With this CLT, students work individually to complete faculty-developed course exams. Once finished, students are able to review and revise their tests within small, collaborative groups. Thus, this CLT allows students to benefit from the shared knowledge base existing within their small, classroom-based peer group. Students in an aural rehabilitation course can take a unit case study-based exam covering aural versus oral approaches to treatment in hearing impaired children. After individually completing their tests, they could work collaboratively, sharing different ideas for each of the exam's case studies. Students could submit individual exams (with changes made after the collaboration indicated in a different color pen/pencil) or could submit a group exam, in which all students in a collaborative group receive the same test grade.

Problem-Based Learning

Problem-based learning (PBL) is a pedagogical method wherein higher level thinking is encouraged when students are asked to analyze problems within small group contexts to form well-conceived solutions. In academic programs in communication sciences and disorders, this technique has obvious merit. Most faculty work to infuse aspects of clinical problem solving into course content, knowing full well that our students, as future clinicians, likely will benefit from practice solving "real life" problems. PBL represents a systematic way to integrate clinical problem solving as one component of creating an active learning environment.

Within the context of PBL, course instructors take on a multifaceted role, one wherein the ability of an instructor to engage students in an active learning process is central to the PBL experience. To this end, Barrows (1992) has stated that:

> The ability of [faculty] to use facilitory teaching skills during the small group learning process is the major determinant of the quality and the success of any educational method aimed at (1) developing students' thinking or reasoning skills (problem solving, metacognition, critical thinking) as they learn, and (2) helping them to become independent, self-directed learners (learning to learn, learning management). (p. 12)

Consistent with the constructivist approach detailed within Chapter 3, Hmelo-Silver and Barrows (2006) suggest that faculty should be collaborators with students, helping to facilitate students' construction of their own learning. This sort of teacher role helps to encourage deep learning through dynamic interactions with students (Mok, Dodd, & Whitehall, 2009). To this end, PBL is considered a teaching strategy "rich in instructional scaffolding" (Schmidt, van der Molen, Winkel, & Wijnen, 2009, p. 238) due to the facilitative responsibilities of teaching in this context. Simply stated, as students work to solve their assigned problem(s), faculty are present as collaborators, asking questions and providing encouragement and support as needed to provide support for students to act as independent thinkers and learners.

Overall, research in the area of PBL would suggest that it is an effective teaching strategy. Consistently, research has found that PBL is a learner-centered approach, which results in better retention of learned information (Dochy, Segers, Van den Bossche, & Gijbels, 2003; Visconti, 2010) and increased knowledge and performance in clinical situations (Baker, McDaniel, Pesut, & Fisher, 2007; Weismer, 2007). Further, other findings would indicate that PBL can help adapt student learning to encourage critical thinking. Schmidt et al. (2009) have found that the use of PBL helps students develop flexible mental models of the world and acts as a valuable tool for "learning how to learn" (p. 229). Additionally, PBL has been associated with increased student engagement and more student time spent on course material (Visconti, 2010).

Although it may sound commonsense to engage CSD students in clinically oriented problem-solving activities, true PBL experiences must be designed carefully. While course instructors act as facilitators of learning as students are addressing the problem(s) to be solved, it is in the consideration of the how the problem will be derived and the task will be executed where care must be taken initially by faculty. Barrows (1992) suggests that any problem-solving group loses its effectiveness with more than seven or eight members, thus creating groups must be accomplished with this in mind. Beyond this, Savery and Duffy (1996) have compiled a list of faculty-centric steps for designing effective PBL experiences that incorporates much of the foundational research into the use of PBL as a teaching technique. Based on their findings, faculty should be mindful of the following when designing PBL experiences (Savery & Duffy, 1996):

1. Learning activities should be presented in a manner anchored to a larger task or problem in a manner that allows students to view their work as valuable for a real-world clinical issue.
2. Support for the learner in developing ownership for the overall problem or task should be facilitated.
3. Problems should be posed in a way that authentic tasks (those that approximate real-life clinical situations or problems) are presented to students in which the cognitive demands placed on the learner are appropriate to the task and context are required.

4. The task and the learning environment should be designed to reflect the complexity of the environment students should be able to function in at the end of the PBL experience.
5. Students should be given ownership of the process used to develop a solution by resisting any impulse to over-proceduralize thinking.
6. The learning environment should be designed to support and challenge the learner's thinking by allowing all valid and reasonable approaches to problem solving to be accessed.
7. Student testing of ideas against alternative views and contexts should be encouraged.
8. Opportunities should be provided for student reflection on both the content learned and the learning process.

The steps outlined previously are those taken by the faculty member seeking to infuse PBL into her teaching. That said, various activities are shown to have efficacy in facilitating higher level thinking and learning in students. The following three steps, consistent with our position that active learning not only engages students but supports learning, outline the cognitive elements of PBL that, when accessed, increase the chances that students will have deep and meaningful learning experiences (Taylor & Miflin, 2008):

1. A problem is posed first, with no specific student preparation necessarily preceding the presentation of the problem.
2. Students activate/articulate existing knowledge as the starting point of discussion in the problem-solving process.
3. Students engage in systematic reasoning about the problem, including applying new learning (p. 756).

We would argue that these different responsibilities could be merged to form one comprehensive set of roles and responsibilities for using PBL in CSD classrooms. Table 6–2 presents our model for PBL. This table combines instructor-centric and student-centric aspects of planning and implementing PBL experiences in a way in which all roles and responsibilities for all stakeholders can be contextualized. Vignette 6–1 provides an example of how PBL can be applied within a CSD course to address a learning need.

Table 6-2. Problem-Based Learning (PBL) Process Roles and Responsibilities

Instructor Roles and Responsibilities	Step #	Student Roles and Responsibilities
Place students into problem-solving groups of (no more than) 5–7 students.	1	
Assign problem for use in PBL process, which is appropriate for students' prior knowledge and current academic needs.	2	
	3	Meet with group. Identify known information related to the assigned problem and then determine what questions remain unanswered/information is needed
	4	Take group informational needs and search for necessary information individually or in groups.
Facilitate student learning by acting as resource to guide problem-solving process.	5	Bring newfound information back to group and share with group mates.
	6	Determine what additional information is needed and then repeat steps 4 and 5 until problem is answered.
	7	Format final reporting of solution(s) to problem as indicated by course instructor.
Provide feedback related to problem-solving process and accuracy of findings.	8	Reflect on the process of solving the problem, determining what worked and what could be handled differently in next PBL context.

Vignette 6–1. Constructing Opportunities for Problem-Based Learning Experiences

Imagine you're a faculty member teaching an undergraduate introduction to an audiology course. In looking at your teaching evaluations from the prior semester, you see that many students commented that you seem to depend on lecture more than collaborative learning experiences. Taking this data to heart, you begin to explore ideas for infusing more opportunities for active learning within your classroom for the coming semester.

You realize that in the past, you've talked about hearing loss and its impact from different perspectives, but have never really let students try to find out about the overall impact of a hearing loss on their own. Understanding the process of setting up PBL experiences following some research into evidence-based educational practices, you decide to set up a PBL experience for your students address the impact of hearing loss for individuals across the age spectrum. The project you envision begins with the following problem that you pose to your students:

> You are an educational audiologist working in your community's local school district. In the course of your daily conversations with teachers and administrators, you realize that few of your colleagues truly understand what a hearing loss is and how it impacts a child's functioning in academic contexts. Your job is to create a brochure/handout that will educate teachers in your school as to the definition, cause, and impact of a hearing loss.

You inform students that they can work with 3–4 peers to complete this task and provide them with several minutes in class to use as initial planning time for this project. You encourage students to use this initial planning time to determine what questions need to be answered and who will seek out relevant information to answer each question. Students spend the next two weeks in and out of class working to complete this project. You remove yourself from lecturing about any topic covered within the scope of this project. You make yourself available for questions, guidance, and support, but refrain from "spoon feeding" students answers to complete this PBL activity. You answer any procedural question that arises, but let the students have the opportunity to construct their own knowledge base for understanding hearing loss and its academic impact. At the conclusion of the PBL experience, you provide students the opportunity to reflect on not only what they've learned, but how they learned it.

Academic Service Learning

Academic Service Learning (ASL) is an approach to teaching that encourages students to apply course-based learning within the community in a way that benefits both students and the community agency involved. Goldberg, Richburg, and Wood (2006) describe ASL as "experiential and reflective problem-based learning in which students enrolled in an academic course provide a needed service to a community partner" (p. 131). Beyond this basic description, we would argue that ASL encourages students to actively apply knowledge acquired though traditional learning means (lectures, reading, etc.) into real-life problem-solving contexts which, in turn, drives the development of higher level thinking skills.

ASL is not a new innovation in higher education, although it has been in the last decade that ASL has caught the attention of faculty as they've searched for ways to encourage civic awareness for their students. Historically, ASL's existence in college-level teaching was observed three-quarters of a century ago in the work of Dewey (1938), who claimed that even in that era, there was a need to link university teaching with community needs.

ASL should not be confused with volunteerism or community service. Rather, ASL differs from those endeavors as a clear intention exists that students and community partners benefit *equally* through involvement with ASL programming (Simons & Cleary, 2006). This is not the case with volunteerism or community service in which the emphasis is on providing a service in return for little personal gain. With ASL, the ideal outcome is realized when community partners have an important need met and students have had the opportunity to apply course content to address real life issues.

ASL projects support student learning in a variety of ways. Vogelgsang and Astin (2000) reported that students engaged in ASL demonstrate better writing skills and higher grade point averages then students not involved in ASL endeavors. Moely, Mercer, Ilustre, Miron, and McFarland (2002) indicated that as a result of ASL experiences, students scored higher on measures of civic engagement and leadership skill acquisition. Other studies have found that ASL helps to increase student appreciation of learning, an increased understanding of how community partners can benefit from collaborative partnerships, increased academic learning, and improved personal/interpersonal development (Goldberg et al, 2006; Simons & Cleary, 2006).

Facilitating Learning via Community-Based Academic Service

Although many researchers have detailed their specific ASL projects and the outcomes from these studies, few actually inform faculty how to design and implement ASL projects of their own. Thus, in this next section we set out to inform readers of concepts that should be at the forefront of any initial ASL project conceptualization, as careful planning from the design phase of any learning project can ensure we meet the needs of our learners.

Direct Versus Indirect Academic Service Learning

Schoenbrodt (2008) described ASL as having both direct and indirect applications, wherein different activities in the process of designing and implementing ASL-related projects can be categorized. This differentiation might be helpful for faculty as part of the process of planning an ASL project and can be explained as follows:

- Indirect service learning is any activity occurring between students and faculty working together to plan for on-site, community-based services or activities that take place away from the community location where any ASL activities are focused. Thus, these indirect service learning activities could take the form of meetings, correspondence, planning materials or project implementation, or any other task that helps set the stage for successful completion of the ASL project within the community.
- Direct service learning is any portion of an ASL activity that occurs during engagement with the community agency involved in the ASL project. Thus, direct service learning is the realization of the ASL project (actual project being implemented within the community), which is a logical outcome resulting from indirect service learning efforts.

Ideally, students engaged in ASL would have the opportunity to be exposed to both direct and indirect service learning opportunities. If the end goal of engaging in ASL is to help students acquire new knowledge across academic and community contexts, then taking part in both the planning for and the implementation of ASL projects are both potentially beneficial exercises for students.

Components of High-Quality Academic Service Learning

Researchers have agreed that ASL is a multidimensional experience, one with a variety of components, which are all critical to a high-quality ASL experience. Thus, it might seem that there might be a "gold standard" for the comprehensive design of ASL projects. That isn't so. Rather, we have a wide body of literature highlighting successful aspects of ASL endeavors. For instance, Goldberg, Richburg, and Wood (2006) have suggested that ASL has four key components that must be addressed. These include the following:

1. Experiential education, which is designed to enhance student learning and teacher effectiveness
2. Establishment of academic achievement and course objectives, which are linked to community service
3. Ongoing and effective student reflection to ensure an understanding of the educational value of ASL work
4. An overriding goal of citizenship, which provides insight into the role of specific disciplines in establishing a healthy community (pp. 131–32)

Similarly, Village (2006) has suggested that four different themes exist which must be attended to in order to provide comprehensive ASL experiences for students:

1. Institutional commitment from colleges and universities to support ASL endeavors on all levels
2. Collaboration to ensure construction of connections amongst faculty, students, and community partners
3. Service that is meaningful to students and community partners
4. Directed student reflection to consider the ASL experience on a personal level (p. 10)

We would posit that these lists of needed ASL components are not yet comprehensive. Although some overlap is evident among the Village (2006) and Goldberg, Richburg, and Wood (2006) models, neither on its own is a true account of the areas to be addressed in ensuring a meaningful, productive ASL experience for students, community partners, or faculty. Rather, we would suggest that by modifying, combining, and adding to various ASL components suggested in prior research, a fully comprehensive model of what ASL should be can be fashioned.

Figure 6–1 outlines the components of ASL we feel to be requisite and comprehensive for a high-quality ASL experience. Notice that these components aren't hierarchical in nature, but rather reflect an interactive relationship among our model's component parts.

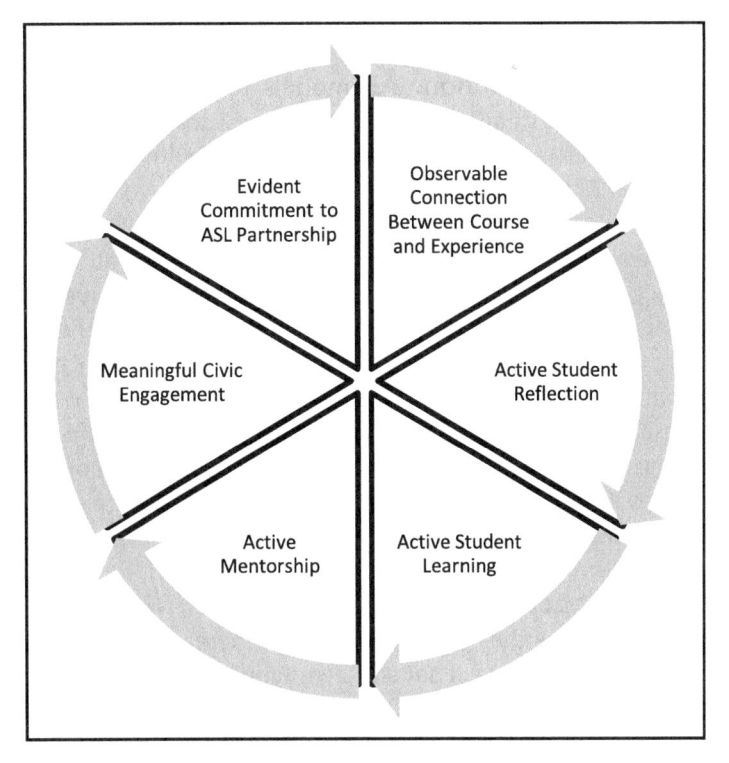

Figure 6–1. Model of requisite components of academic service learning.

This is endemic to the design and understanding of our view of ASL as we believe that the interaction of these aspects of ASL is what drives successful learning experiences within a community context.

We have suggested six distinct components for our ASL model, each of which is explained in the following sections.

Observable Connection between Course and Experience. Although this might seem like a very evident component for ASL, the need for a clear, observable connection between the course a student is enrolled in and any ASL experience within that course cannot be underscored enough. ASL functions to extend learning in a different sort of classroom: the community. Thus, faculty working to integrate ASL opportunities within their courses must be very thoughtful in their planning to ensure an integrated experience between classroom-based learning and community-based application of this learning.

Active Student Reflection. All models for ASL education that we've encountered detail the need for active student reflection as an integral part of any ASL experience (Goldberg, Richburg, and Wood, 2006; Simons & Cleary, 2006; Village, 2006). And, we would agree that this is a very valuable component for learning through community-based service. Chapter 3 of this text detailed at length the importance of reflection as a vehicle to drive real cognitive change. Reflection allows for meta-cognitive self-reflection on the part of students, which can help in the construction of personal meaning from their ASL experience(s). Faculty members choosing to support opportunities for student reflection do so with the understanding that students who make connections amongst class and community experiences are more likely to realize the value of their experiences in ASL as being academically and civically relevant.

Active Student Learning. Few faculty members would engage in ASL projects unless they were certain that increased student learning was a likely outcome. That said, we would support the need for student involvement in any ASL project to be as active in nature as possible to ensure that students are able to make meaningful connections between their academic learning and relevant personal experiences. Research has indicated that students actively engaged in problem solving have an increased sense of ownership in the learning process and are able to develop higher-level thinking skills experientially within a meaningful context (Zlotkowski, 2001).

Active Mentorship. ASL projects provide a very rich environment for professional mentoring. Faculty and community partners engaged in ASL projects are able to engage with students in a manner not evident in classroom-based learning environments. Due to the applied nature of most ASL projects, faculty have the opportunity to bridge the theory-to-practice gap often evident in our classroom-based instruction. In doing so, faculty can guide emerging clinicians, assist in the solving of "real-life" problems in a practical setting, and develop relationships with students who aren't as vocally engaged within the typical classroom environment. Mentoring relationships developed as a part of ASL have the potential to sustain themselves over time, which can drive other projects and additional student learning. Chapter 8 provides additional information related to mentoring of students.

Meaningful Civic Engagement. Although we certainly understand that "meaning" can be a subjective judgment, we feel that there should be a direct and easily observable benefit for any proposed ASL project for both students and community partners. By this, we mean that ASL projects should provide an "appreciable" (Ginsberg, 2007, p. 6) benefit for a particular community partner while resulting in a clearly observable outcome for students. In support of this notion, Simons and Cleary (2006) suggest that any ASL project undertaken should have a short-term timeframe so that students are able to observe the impact of their efforts for a given community group.

Evident Commitment to ASL Partnership. Work toward the completion of ASL projects cannot seem like an afterthought to the completion of a given course. Rather, we would urge faculty who design ASL projects to integrate work for their community partners throughout the semester, to the greatest extent possible. Students who are able to observe collaborative relationships modeled between faculty and community partners are more likely to engage in such community-based efforts throughout their professional careers (Payne, 2000). Thus, the need for faculty to commit to community partnerships is clear.

Vignette 6–2 outlines one way ASL can be used to compliment classroom-based teaching. Beyond the components we've provided for guidance in the creation of ASL experiences for students, we have additional suggestions for faculty looking to engage in ASL projects to support the implementation of any CSD course:

1. Find novel ways to make the community your classroom. Seek out opportunities for your students to involve themselves in community-wide efforts to improve conditions for individuals and their families with speech, language, or hearing impairments.
2. Keep current with published research literature related to ASL and civic engagement in clinically based fields of study to determine the most meaningful methods for engaging in community-based learning. The information we've offered here provides the foundation for conceptualizing the scope and impact of ASL. That said, new studies are published frequently containing new approaches to ASL, innovations for execution of new ASL projects, and efficacy data, which provides an expanding evidence-based for effective ASL design and implementation.
3. Investigate methods of securing funding from various funding sources to support the implementation and execution of community-based learning projects.

Technology for Engaged Learning

Technology has been the driving force behind the globalization of markets, both financial and academic. Hazari, North, and Moreland (2009) stated that "as technology continues to become commonly used for global communication and productivity, technology skills must be incorporated by educators in the delivery of curriculum content" (p. 187). Concurrent with these views are findings from research that suggest that not only does the use of technology help to motivate students, but it can promote active student learning within the classroom (Schrand, 2008).

Vignette 6–2. Constructing Opportunities for Academic Service Learning Projects

Imagine you are teaching a language disorders course for graduate students in speech-language pathology at your university. After reading literature related to ASL, you feel that your class would benefit from involvement with a community-based service project, and after having several conversations with personal contacts within the community to determine which potential community partner was the best match for your ASL project, you were able to structure a plan in which your entire graduate class would be able to take part in a project aimed at preventing language impairments an "at-risk" population of low-income preschool-aged children. The plan you develop has the following components:

- All students in your course would be randomly assigned to one of four groups. Each group was to work collaboratively to plan an hour-long workshop for parents of low-income preschool-aged children that fit into the theme for the semester: "Using Storybooks to Help Your Child Learn." Specific topics to be covered by the four groups of students were chosen: the importance of reading books with young children, teaching new vocabulary using storybooks, teaching rhyming using storybooks, and facilitating written language development using storybooks. Each topic would be assigned to each group, ensuring comprehensive coverage of topics throughout the semester. Under your plan, one topic would be presented each month to parents over the course of the semester. Each of these presentations would correspond to the time in class when these topics were being covered, so as to extend learning beyond the classroom into the community. Workshops were required to provide information about each topic and ideas/suggestions/techniques for parents to use when reading books with their children.
- As part of each workshop, students were to be responsible for developing a brief handout for parents providing good, practical advice using parent-friendly language to explain the importance of each topic. Students also would need to provide information for families to assist in gaining access to children's books at little to no cost.

continues

Vignette 6–2. *continued*

> - It was mandatory that each workshop would provide an opportunity for parents to practice the techniques and strategies being discussed within the workshop, so students will need to plan for practical application of their material as part of their planning process.
> - Students will prepare a list of "take home ideas" for parents to facilitate future use of workshop ideas, including book lists, community resources, etc.
> - Each group will meet with you weekly to update progress and share successes and questions the group might have as a result of their work together.
> - Throughout the semester, students would complete a series of reflective papers to indicate their perceptions and impressions relative to their experiences and how those experiences furthered their understanding of clinical work and course-specific learning.
>
> Thus, the indirect service learning components of this project would be comprised of efforts to plan for the implementation of your ASL project and included group meetings to plan for all project components, research needed for each group's specific topic, the generation of take home ideas, planning for each workshop, and coordination with the community partner at various junctures over the course of the semester. Direct service learning will be realized through the actual delivery of the workshop to parents, the demonstration of techniques to encourage carryover of new skills for families in attendance, and the dissemination of information for future use by families in attendance.

Fortunately, many avenues exist for faculty to pursue to infuse different technologies into their teaching. From options that allow for courses to be delivered entirely over the Internet via online teaching and learning, to the use of various tools such as clickers or podcasting, the buffet of options faculty can choose from is plentiful. The trick is choosing from the available options with purpose and care. We have observed faculty using technology just for the sake of using technology, rather than to meet a specific educational need. To this end, we would emphasize that technology should dovetail with the educational goals a faculty member is seeking to achieve;

use of technology should not itself be the goal. By this, we mean that any technology used should be selected based on the value it might add to learning, rather than the cache it might offer to the faculty member or students involved in a particular education experience. Because, unless you're teaching about a technology specific to the diagnosis or treatment of a communication-based disorder (e.g., hearing aid technology or videostroboscopy), the technology that you use as part of your teaching isn't the point. It's the complement to your teaching that can assist in engaging your students to facilitate active engagement and drive increased learning.

The following section highlights a few technologies currently demonstrated to have a positive impact on student learning.

Internet-Based Teaching and Learning

Over the last two decades, the use of the Internet to support faculty throughout the implementation of a course's curriculum has steadily increased, as have the options for how the Internet can guide the learning process. In addition to traditional, in-person courses, contemporary colleges and universities generally offer some courses in an entirely Internet-based (online) format, as well as some that are taught in a hybrid manner (a mixture of traditional, in-person teaching and some component of Internet-based learning). Faculty have many different platforms (e.g., Blackboard, Sakai) available for use in organizing and delivering Internet-based course content and have the advantage that many (if not most) students are familiar with the Internet and have few difficulties in accessing any course content delivered in an online format.

Palloff and Pratt (1999) derived "definitional elements of online education" (p. 16) which, in our view, are central to understanding the basis for how online learning can be considered and include the following:

- Separation of instructor and learner in time and place for some part of the instructional process
- Faculty-student (or student-student) connection via various educational media
- Volitional control of the learning process resting with the learner

Our interest in these characteristics of online education are particularly piqued by the third bulleted item as it indicates a need for students to be actively involved in constructing their own learning. As strong advocates for active learning practices in higher education, we realize their value as part of the teaching and learning process. When considering Internet-based learning, we feel that the need to promote active participation is even more focused as students are tasked with organizing, managing, and constructing their own learning experiences as part of most online classes. They have to have a sense for what needs to be done and how it should be accomplished and must do this independent of any traditional course support structure. Due in large part to this need for active involvement as part of Internet-based coursework, researchers have found that students in online courses are more reflective, spend more time preparing for class by completing readings and outside research, and generally are more involved in class discussions (Rabe-Hemp, Woollen, & Humiston, 2009). For more discussion regarding structuring active, engaged learning in an online or hybrid format class, see Chapter 5.

As research has demonstrated a positive relationship between using Internet-based instruction and both student engagement and learning outcomes (Chen, Lambert, & Guidry, 2010), the use and implementation of online teaching and learning remains a viable choice faculty can make to design high-quality learning experiences. That said, we feel that faculty should keep several notions supported by EBE research in mind when considering the creation of hybrid or entirely online courses. First and foremost, if students aren't comfortable, they will not participate (Rocca, 2010). Students need to feel at ease in online class settings. Using humor, having an interest in students as individuals, and recruiting students' interest in becoming involved in class discussions are all methods that increase students' comfort with an Internet-based class. It is also important to note that multiple communication channels may be related to higher levels of student engagement (Dixson, 2010). The more modalities you can access as a faculty member to communicate with (and reach!) your students, the better off your students will be. Finally, student-to-student and instructor-to-student communication are correlated with higher levels of student engagement within the context of Internet-based courses (Dixson, 2010; Rabe-Hemp, Woollen, & Humiston, 2009). With this in mind, communication in online course settings is not a one-way street. Both students and course instructors need to have the opportunity to interact and communicate with one another in order to build a sense of community, to build collaborative partnerships, and to demonstrate interaction amongst all stakeholders in online teaching and learning.

With regard to discussions, online threaded discussions are a successful vehicle for promoting the building of collaborative and information sharing skills (Schoenarcher, 2009). Online discussions should be connected by topic wherever possible in order to assist students in drawing connections among postings, as well as to allow for a space where knowledge is applied in a trial-and-error fashion over the course of a semester. Additionally, asynchronous discussion methods yield more time for students to use in order to thoughtfully consider content prior to becoming engaged (Rabe-Hemp et al., 2009). Students often prefer more processing time to consider different angles for various questions/content than is provided in traditional in-person courses. The ability for students to read a question, ponder it, and answer it at their convenience (as is typical for many online courses and is assumed within the use of the term "asynchronous") provides students with an advantage, wherein they can derive the quality of the question and respond in a manner totally consistent with their own schedules, needs, and preferences. Finally, when students act as facilitators of online discussions, other students are more likely to post contributions in online discussion forums (Poole, 2000).

Podcasting

Podcasting is a technology that, while available for use for many years, has just recently been identified as a technological option for course instructors to enhance communication with students. The recent jump in the use of educationally based podcasting is easy to attribute to various technological advances as podcasts are "easy to use across multiple environments, typical over computer speakers, a car stereo, and over headphones" (Campbell, 2005, p. 34). Individuals between the ages of 18–29 constitute the largest group of podcasting users in the United States and beyond, indicating that traditional college students might well be the best and most able users of this technology (Pew Research, 2008).

Podcasting uses streaming and downloadable audio files to share information with others with ease. Podcasts can be created by anyone with an interest in sharing audio files. Interested users can simply record an audio file using a digital voice recorder and then upload the recorded audio file to a computer. Podcasts can be edited easily using free or low-cost editing software and then uploaded for others to listen to. Finalized podcasts can be uploaded to a Website, which allows potential listeners to subscribe to various podcasts (e.g., iTunes) or can simply be shared via email or posted to course management Web sites (e.g., Blackboard or Sakai). Students easily can access these files and listen to them in a manner most comfortable to their own technological know-how. Podcasting has been described as a technology only limited by society's collective imagination (Bull, 2005).

While used to convey information and provide entertainment to listeners, use of podcasting as an educational tool within clinically based academic programs is on the rise, as podcasting is developing a more visible profile as a relevant, appropriate way to disseminate information and create networks of professional learners (Friberg, 2008; Maag, 2006; Rowell, Corl, Johnson, & Fishman, 2006). In fact, within the fields of speech-language pathology and audiology, ASHA embraced podcasting as an effective method to use for providing continuing education opportunities and delivering information to students and consumers of clinically-based speech, language, and/or hearing services (Kuster, 2007).

Most research on the use of podcasting would suggest that podcasting alone doesn't positively impact student learning, although the use of podcasts can help students when used as a supplemental tool for supporting mastery of course concepts and for promoting student engagement and faculty/student communication (Friberg, 2008; Lonn & Teasley, 2009). Along these lines, Fernandez, Simo and Sallan (2009) studied the efficacy of podcasting and have suggested the following guidelines as being part of a "framework of principles for good practice in higher education:" (p. 385)

- Podcasting is a powerful tool that acts as a complement for supporting the delivery and understanding of course content and should act as a wholesale replacement of traditional teaching practices.
- The use of podcasting helps students to perceive a sort of permanent contact between students and faculty, which has the benefit of increasing students' motivation to learn and interact.
- Podcasting allows for students to access course information in a diverse manner, supporting the need for multimodal instructional practices to best engage students in learning.

In order to capitalize on these principles, course instructors might choose to use podcasts to supplement course instruction in a variety of ways. Figure 6–2 provides a brief listing of ideas which can be used as a starting point for podcasting in the classroom.

To Address Procedural Needs	To Address Communication Needs	To Address Learning Needs
• provide information relative to the format of the class, including calendar or syllabus review updates to ensure students have all the information they need to proceed successfully with course content for the week	• disseminate student projects/presentations for peers or for other groups of individuals • record interviews with practicing clinicians related to relevant areas of professional practice for given courses	• provide exam review information/sessions for students to download and access at their leisure • provide examples of aspects of the assessment process, including: exemplar interviews, language sample collections, vocal assessments, fluency assessments, etc. • provide summaries of journal articles germane to course content for students to access for review of applied or basic research

Figure 6–2. Potential uses for podcasting in the classroom.

Clickers

Clickers are referred to by a variety of names, such as electronic student response systems, personal response systems, or zappers. Clickers resemble remote controls and are used by students in educational environments to provide feedback in situ, that is, during real-time course activities. Course instructors can pose questions, typically in a multiple choice or Likert-type scale format, which can be interspersed as individual slides within a PowerPoint presentation or can be presented as questions separate from a more formal presentation/lecture. Course instructors can use commercially available software packages (e.g., Turning Point) to facilitate this process.

Students view these questions on a projector screen, and then press a button on their clicker to indicate an answer selection and results are tabulated and displayed for the course instructor within seconds. Results are available for faculty and can be presented to students for their viewing, as well. Using this sort of format, course instructors are provided with immediate data reflecting students' comprehension of new concepts or perceptions/attitudes related to a particular issue (Kolikant, Drane, & Calkins, 2010). Kenwright (2009) suggests that clickers can be most effectively used for answering questions, completing quizzes and self assessments, and performing course evaluations. Faculty have also reported that clickers can be used effectively to discuss sensitive information or issues that typically yield few students willing to publically discuss their feelings, attitudes, or beliefs.

As was the case with podcasting, the use of clickers alone has not been proven to increase student learning, although it has been found that students perceive that they understand course concepts better and earn better exam grades when using clickers (Prather & Brissenden, 2009). Rather, most research has focused on the affective implications of the use of clicker technologies on student participation, engagement, and overall support for active learning. Within these parameters, data has demonstrated that clickers are effective technological supplements to traditional in-course teaching, which serve as tools to engage and motivate students (Kolikant et al., 2010). Data also would suggest that the use of clickers also leads to improved student attendance in class and increased participation in class discussions (Kenwright, 2009).

As was discussed earlier in Chapter 3, active learning allows for students to act as constructionists in developing their individual understanding of course content. While this is certainly true and we would encourage faculty to strive to actively involve their students in all aspects of teaching and learning, there will likely still be students in any class we teach who simply are uncomfortable with letting others know their views or perspectives related to a particular topic for myriad reasons. One benefit to the instant feedback provided for faculty when clickers are used in the classroom is that students are able to express their views with complete anonymity, which can alleviate a major roadblock to student participation in class: the possibility that students might be judged as being unintelligent or different from their peers (Martyn, 2007; Stowell, Oldham, & Bennett, 2010). Beyond this fear, Bransford, Brophy, and Williams (2000) identified three other student-centered characteristics, which might discourage students from participating in class discussions. These characteristics, along with Kolikant, Drane, and Calkin's (2010) suggestions as to how the use of clickers can help work around these participation roadblocks are detailed in Table 6–3.

Martyn (2007) summarizes "best practices" for faculty to be mindful of as they implement the use of clickers within a given class setting. These best practices have been compiled from a variety of sources and include eighteen suggestions for course instructors. We've culled this list to eight suggestions, as we feel that these are the most important considerations for faculty using clickers as a supplemental classroom technology. Our selected suggestions include the following (Martyn, 2007):

1. *Do not make the questions you ask for students to answer overly complex.* Rather, design questions that have the potential to lead to discussion about various course topics.
2. *Allow sufficient time for students to answer questions using their clickers.* Students need to feel that they have "thinking time" in order to consider their answers. Suggested time ranges for allowing responses via clicker range from 15–30 seconds.
3. *Allow time for discussion between questions.* Clickers have efficacy for use in higher education because of their affective impact. Students are more likely to actively engage with the course content you're trying to cover if you allow for discussion

Table 6–3. Potential Benefits of Clickers As a Method of Increasing Student Participation

	Characteristics that discourage students from conversing during lecture-based classes[1]:	Ways in which use of clickers might counteract conversational drawbacks in lecture-based classes[2]:
1	Students are not aware of their own difficulties understanding or applying course content.	Students can assess their own learning and comprehension by using clickers.
2	Students don't know what it is they're struggling to understand.	Immediate feedback allows students to view errors, and they can (possibly) observe that others made similar mistakes.
3	Students feel isolated, as if they are the only ones struggling to assimilate new information or content.	Anonymous feedback/results can alleviate anxiety about looking less intelligent than peers within the class.

[1]Bransford, Brophy, and Williams (2000).
[2]Kolikant, Drane, and Calkins (2010).

between questions, rather than rushing from one question to the next.

4. *Encourage active discussion with the students who constitute your audience.* Faculty should strive to pose questions for students to address using clickers which have potential to segue into rich, cooperative discussions. Factually-based questions can be posed, but as they don't always lead to much dialogue. Therefore, we would encourage faculty to vary the type of questions they ask students to answer using clickers. Inclusion of opinion or perception-based questions often will lead to active class discussions.

5. *Position questions to be answered via clicker at periodic intervals throughout the class period.* Strategic planning for using clickers across a course session is important. If clickers are truly being used to spur discussion and increase affective aspects of

learning, faculty should try to balance the use of clickers across a course meeting to ensure that questions aren't ill-spaced within a class meeting.
6. *Do not ask too many questions; use them for specific points you want to emphasize for knowledge or discussion.* Choose which points in your class period are most critical and design clicker-based questions around those points. Using clickers to answer too many questions might easily dilute the purpose you hope to achieve by using this supplemental technology in the first place.
7. *Provide clear instructions on how to use clickers to your students.* Mediate the process of using clickers with your students. Tell them why you're using them and what purpose you hope they will serve pedagogically speaking. Make sure students understand not only how to use the hardware (clicker), but how their feedback will be illustrated and interpreted to avoid any confusion for students.
8. *Do not over-use clickers, or they might lose their potential to engage students in the learning process.* Over-use of clickers is similar to over-use of any specific teaching strategy. Students will lose interest in it, and its effectiveness will wane. To maximize the impact of clickers, strategic planning is helpful to ensure appropriate, functional use of this technology.

We view clickers as a technology that would be fairly easy to incorporate into just about any CSD course. Consider the following options:

- In an audiology course in which students are debating the ethics of hearing aid dispensing, students could be asked to assign a value on a Likert-type scale that reflects their perceptions as to whether or not online hearing aid dispensing is an ethical practice.
- Students in a graduate phonology course could be asked to rank their treatment priorities for a child with unintelligible speech.
- Students in a graduate dysphagia course could be asked to interpret a videofluroscopic swallow study and indicate the phase of swallowing where aspiration was noted.

Note that with each of these examples, students could assess their perception(s) without fear of being "wrong" in front of their peers.

And, in each example, the potential for rich discussion of student answers exists. These questions would exemplify our interpretation of clicker use as being a springboard for active learning.

Wikis

Wikis are shared Web sites that allow users to report and edit information in an asynchronous manner. Generally, wikis are comprised of Web pages that are edited by any user to house an ever-changing compendium of data focused on a particular topic or topics. In order to allow for the rapid evolution of information, wikis access "Web 2.0," which allows users to use the Internet interactively, rather than passively. Hazari, North, and Moreland (2009) state that Web 2.0 allows "users [to] add information to the Web environment in which they interact with other interested members" (p. 187). Leuf and Cunningham (2001) characterize the creation of wikis as being an ongoing process of collaboration and creation, which constantly changes the content of the wiki itself. Additionally, wikis have been characterized as being simple, flexible, and open (Su & Beaumont, 2010), allowing for students to interact via online processes, which are collaborative and interactive in nature. The use of wikis is associated closely with the social-constructivist educational philosophy, which encourages a student-driven, teacher-facilitated evolution of learning (Su & Beaumont, 2010).

How are wikis used in education? We've found that wikis are used in a variety of ways to meet myriad curricular needs:

- To construct reflection journals
- To complete a research project or proposal
- To compile a summary of readings (e.g., chapters, research articles)
- To produce or complete study guides
- To produce or populate glossaries with course-specific terminology
- To manage group work within a given project context
- To use as a tool for brainstorming
- To make lists for class, projects, etc.
- To generate a collection of Web links to important organizations, information, data, or community agency

These wiki uses easily could be adapted for application in many CSD courses. It would be possible to create a wiki to facilitate the development of a listing of Web links for professional certification on national, state and regional levels for students in a professional issues course. Audiology students in an assessment course could create a wiki to inform potential patients and community members how to read and interpret the results of an audiogram. Students in a vocal disorders course could use a wiki to plan for efforts to provide education to singers to reduce vocal abuse and strain.

Foord (2007) developed an acronym, STOLEN, to represent the six components of wiki use that are likely to increase the chances of successful use and implementation of wikis to support and drive student learning. Each component of the STOLEN is outlined in Figure 6–3.

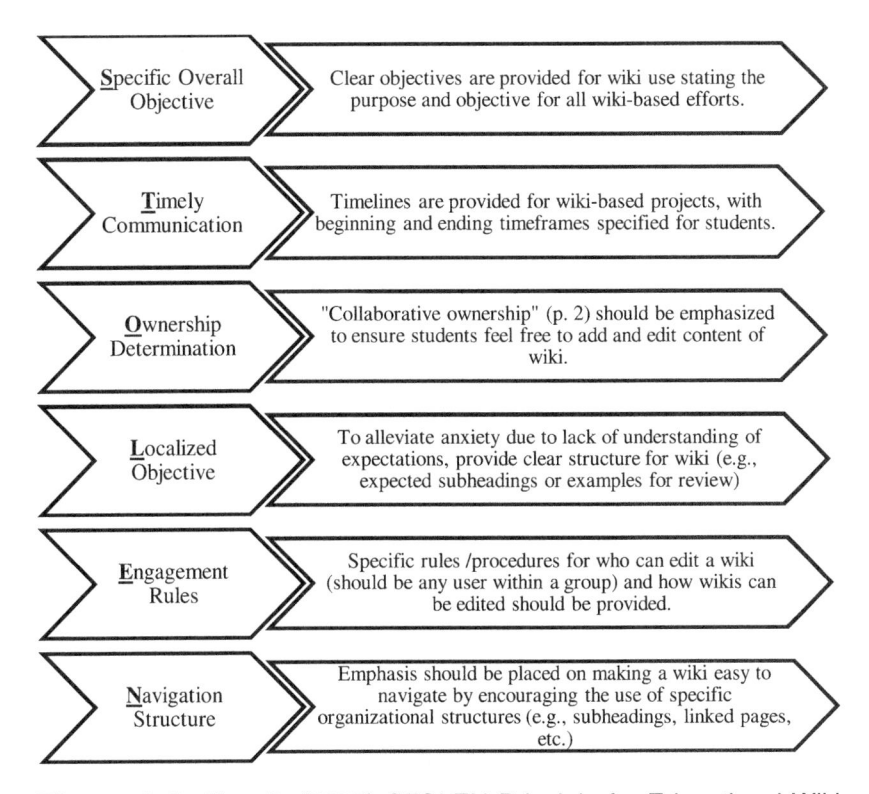

Specific Overall Objective	Clear objectives are provided for wiki use stating the purpose and objective for all wiki-based efforts.
Timely Communication	Timelines are provided for wiki-based projects, with beginning and ending timeframes specified for students.
Ownership Determination	"Collaborative ownership" (p. 2) should be emphasized to ensure students feel free to add and edit content of wiki.
Localized Objective	To alleviate anxiety due to lack of understanding of expectations, provide clear structure for wiki (e.g., expected subheadings or examples for review)
Engagement Rules	Specific rules/procedures for who can edit a wiki (should be any user within a group) and how wikis can be edited should be provided.
Navigation Structure	Emphasis should be placed on making a wiki easy to navigate by encouraging the use of specific organizational structures (e.g., subheadings, linked pages, etc.)

Figure 6–3. Foord's (2007) STOLEN Principle for Educational Wiki Use.

Each of the principles discussed as part of the STOLEN model support increased levels of student engagement, making the use of wiki technology in this manner potentially impactful in increasing active learning for students. By being specific with objectives, timely in providing expectations and feedback, allowing students ownership of their work, setting flexible rules, and encouraging organized outcomes, wikis allow students to drive their own learning within teacher-driven parameters.

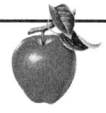

Vignette 6–3. Applying Technology to Your Teaching

Suppose that you're a CSD faculty member teaching a course on professional issues in speech-language pathology and audiology. And, because you feel that the content of your course is amenable to online delivery, you choose to teach this course in an entirely online format. You design your course, create your syllabus, and teach it for the first time over the course of a regular academic semester. At the conclusion of the semester, you feel as though the course was fairly successful, but you want to ascertain what the students thought about the course and its online format.

To accomplish this, you invited five students, each of whom were enrolled in your course, to form an informal focus group, which would provide a form of summative evaluation of the entire course. Specifically, when the focus group convened, you asked students to share their view of the most positive and negative aspects of their course experience. While indicating that the course was well implemented and designed, focus-group participants indicated that they missed the personal, anecdotal stories and information that typically accompanies course lecture and delivery in more traditional, in-person courses. Focus-group members felt that having access to these stories and anecdotes would help future students to develop a framework

Vignette 6–3. *continued*

for recalling course information while simultaneously making course content richer with "real world" contextual support.

Using results from the focus group, you do a bit of research and determined that my students were not alone, that in fact, the opinions of my students mirrored earlier research that found students in online courses desired more auditory feedback, preferring to augment their readings and online asynchronous discussions with stories detailing the experiences and perspectives of others. Taking this information into account, you began to consider ways in which you could augment your course content to increase student engagement and overall retention of information. During this search, you came across information related to the use of podcasting in higher education. Podcasting allows for students to access prepared audio files, which can be downloaded to students' computers or MP3 players. Although not commonplace in university-level departments of speech-language pathology and audiology, podcasting has been used to improve teaching and further engage students in the learning process. Podcasting seemed a tremendous fit for your particular pedagogical needs.

As such, you acquired the basic recording equipment needed to begin to record podcasts for your students, and you developed a series of six topic areas you thought would be complimentary to course content as the basis for my course podcasts. You felt that these podcasts successfully would infuse real-life examples from other practicing professionals as a supplemental to the materials already being utilized as a part of my course. Each podcast featured a different speech-language pathologist or audiologist being interviewed about their experiences germane their professional practice, as related to each of the six topic areas. The recordings from each interview was edited and saved as a separate podcast. These podcasts would be made available to students in the next time you taught the course in question. Following the conclusion of the first semester in which podcasts were available for students' use, you develop a plan to survey students to determine whether the podcasts were effective in providing a real-world perspective for students relative to course topics and made adjustments, as needed.

References

Baker, C. M., McDaniel, A. M., Pesut, D. J., & Fisher, M. L. (2007). Learning skills profiles of masters students in nursing administration: Assessing the impact of problem-based learning. *Nursing Education Perspectives, 28*(4), 190–195.

Barkley, E., Cross, K., & Major, C. (2005). *Collaborative learning techniques: A handbook for college faculty.* San Francisco, CA: Jossey-Bass.

Barrows, H. (1992). *The tutorial process.* Springfield, IL: Southern Illinois University School of Medicine.

Bransford, J., Brophy, S., & Williams, S. (2000). When computer technologies meet the learning sciences: Issues and opportunities. *Journal of Applied Developmental Psychology, 21*(1), 59–84.

Bull, G. (2005, November). Podcasting and the long tail [Electronic version]. *Learning and Leading with Technology, 33*, 24–25.

Campbell, G. (2005, November/December). There's something in the air: Podcasting in education [Electronic version]. Educause Review. Retrieved from http://www.educause.edu/EDUCAUSE+Review/EDUCAUSEReviewMagazineVolume40/TheresSomethingintheAirPodcast/158014

Chen, D., Lambert, A. & Guidry, K. (2010). Engaging online learners: The impact of web-based learning technology on college student engagement. *Computers and Education, 54*(4), 1222–1232.

Christiansen, B., & Jensen, K. (2008). Emotional learning within the framework of nursing education. *Nursing Education in Practice, 8*(5), 328–334.

Davis, B. (1993). *Tools for teaching.* San Francisco, CA: Jossey-Bass.

Dewey, J. (1938). *Experience and education.* New York, NY: Collier.

Dixson, M. (2010). Creating effective student engagement in online courses: What do students find engaging. *Journal of the Scholarship of Teaching and Learning, 10*(2), 1–13.

Dochy, F., Segers, M., Van den Bossche, P., & Gijbels, D. (2003). Effects of problem-based learning: A meta-analysis. *Learning and Instruction, 13*(5), 533–568.

Ezzedeen, S. (2008). Facilitating class discussion around current and controversial issues: Ten recommendations for teachers. *College Teaching, 56*(4), 230–236.

Fernandez, V., Simo, P., & Sallan, J. (2009). Podcasting: A new technological tool to facilitate good practice in higher education. *Computers & Education, 53*(2), 385–392.

Foord, D. (2007). The STOLEN principle for using wikis educationally. Retrieved from http://www.a6training.co.uk/resources/STOLEN ticksheet.doc.

Friberg, J. (2008). The use of supplemental podcasting as an instructional tool in an online classroom setting. *Issues in Higher Education, 11*(2), 61–66.

Fritschner, L. (2000). Inside the undergraduate college classroom: Faculty and students differ on the meaning of student participation. *Journal of Higher Education, 71*, 342–362.

Ginsberg, S. (2007). Academic service learning in speech-language pathology and audiology education. *Issues in Higher Education, 10*, 6–8.

Goldberg, L., Richburg, C., & Wood, L. (2006). Active learning though service learning. *Communication Disorders Quarterly, 27*(3), 131–145.

Hazari, S., North, A., & Moreland, D. (2009). Investigating pedagogical value of wiki technology. *Journal of Informational Systems Education, 20*(2), 187–198.

Hmelo-Silver, C., & Barrows, H. (2006). Goals and strategies of a problem-based learning facilitator. *The Interdisciplinary Journal of Problem-based Learning, 1*(1), 21–39.

Kenwright, K. (2009). Clickers in the classroom. *TechTrends: Linking Research and Practice to Improve Learning, 53*(1), 74–77.

Kolikant, Y., Drane, D., & Calkins, S. (2010). "Clickers" as catalysts for transformation of teachers. *College Teaching, 58*, 127–135.

Kuster, J. (2007). Professional—and personal—podcasting. *The ASHA Leader, 12*(16), 24–25.

Leuf, B., & Cunningham, W. (2001). *The wiki way: Quick collaboration on the web.* Redwood City, CA: Addison-Wesley Professional.

Loke, A., & Chow, F. (2007). Learning partnership—the experience of peer tutoring among nursing students: A qualitative study. *International Journal of Nursing Studies, 44*(2), 237–244.

Lonn, S., & Teasley, S. (2009). Podcasting in higher education: What are the implications for teaching and learning? *Internet and Higher Education, 12*(2), 88–92.

Maag, M. (2006). Podcasting and mp3 players: Emerging educational technologies. *Computers Informatics Nursing, 24*(1), 9–12.

Maeroff, G. (2003). *A classroom of one: How online education is changing our schools and colleges.* New York, NY: Palgrave Macmillian.

Martyn, M. (2007). Clickers in the classroom: An active learning approach. *Educause Quarterly, 30*(2). Retrieved from http://www.educause.edu/EDUCAUSE+Quarterly/EDUCAUSEQuarterlyMagazineVolum/ClickersintheClassroomAnActive/157458

McKeachie, W. (1999). *Teaching tips: Strategies, research and theory for college and university teachers* (10th ed.). Boston, MA: Houghton Mifflin.

Moely, B., Mercer, S., Ilustre, D., Miron, D., & McFarland, M. (2002). Psychometric properties and correlates of the civic attitudes and skills questionnaire (CASQ): A measure of student's attitudes related to service learning. *Michigan Journal of Community Service Learning, 8*(2), 15–26.

Mok, C., Dodd, B., & Whitehill, T. (2009). Speech-language pathology students' approaches to learning in a problem-based curriculum. *International Journal of Speech-Language Pathology, 11*(6), 472–481.

Palloff, R., & Pratt, K. (1999). *Building learning communities in cyberspace: Effective strategies for the online classroom.* San Francisco:, CA Jossey Bass.

Payne, D. (2000). *Evaluating service-learning activities & programs.* Lanham, MD: The Scarecrow Press.

Pew Research. (2008). *Pew Internet Project Data Memo.* Washington DC: Author.

Poole, D. (2000). Student participation in a discussion-oriented outline course: A case study. *Journal of Research on Computing in Education, 33*, 162–177.

Prather, E., & Brissenden, G. (2009). Clickers as data gathering tools and students' attitudes, motivations, and beliefs on their use in this application. *Astronomy Education Review, 8*(1). Retrieved from http://aer.aas.org/resource/1/aerscz/v8/i1/p010103_s1

Rabe-Hemp, C., Woollen, S., & Humiston, G. (2009). A comparative analysis of student engagement, learning and satisfaction in lecture halls and online settings. *Quarterly Review of Distance Education, 10*(2), 207–218.

Rocca, K. (2010). Student participation in the college classroom: An extended multidisciplinary literature review. *Communication Education, 59*(2), 185–213.

Roehling, P., Vander Kooi, T., Dykema, S., Quisenberry, B., & Vandlen, C. (2011). Engaging the millennial generation in class discussions. *College Teaching, 59*, 1–6.

Rowell, M., Corl, F., Johnson, P., & Fishman, E. (2006). Internet-based dissemination of educational audiocasts: A primer in podcasting—how to do it. *American Journal of Roentgenology, 186*, 1792–1796.

Savery, J., & Duffy, T. (1996). Problem based learning: An instructional model and its constructivist framework. In B. Wilson (Ed.), *Constructivist learning environments: Case studies in instructional design* (pp. 135–148). Englewood Cliffs, NJ: Educational Technology.

Schmidt, H., van der Molen, H., Winkel, W., & Wijnen, W. (2009). Constructivist, problem-based learning does work: A meta-analysis of curricular comparisons involving a single medical school. *Educational Psychology, 44*(4), 227–249.

Schoenarcher, S. (2009). Building online capital through online class discussions: A little freedom goes a long way. *Journal of Educational Technology Systems, 37*(3), 291–303.

Schoenbrodt, L. (2008). Service learning 201: Beyond the basics. *Issues in Higher Education, 11*(1), 36–40.

Schrand, T. (2008). Tapping into active learning and multiple intelligences with interactive media: A low-threshold classroom approach. *College Teaching, 56*(20), 78–84.

Simons, L., & Cleary, B. (2006). The influence of service learning on students' personal and social development. *College Teaching 54*, 307–319.

Smith, D., (1977). College classroom interactions and critical thinking. *Journal of Educational Psychology, 69*(2), 180-190.

Stowell, J., Oldham, T., & Bennett, D. (2010). Using student response systems ("clickers") to conformity and shyness. *Teaching of Psychology, 37*, 135–140.

Su, F., & Beaumont, C. (2010). Evaluating the use of a wiki for collaborative learning. *Innovations in Education and Teaching International, 47*(4), 417–431.

Taylor, D. & Miflin, B. (2008). Problem-based learning: Where are we now? *Medical Teacher, 30*(8), 742-763.

Village, D. (2006). Qualities of effective service learning in physical therapist education. *Journal of Physical Therapy Education, 20*(3), 8–17.

Visconti, C. (2010). Problem-based learning: Teaching skills for evidence-based practice. *Perspectives on Issues in Higher Education, 13*(1), 27–31.

Vogelgsang, L., & Astin, A. (2000). Comparing the effects of community service and service learning. *Michigan Journal of Community Service Learning, 7*, 25–34.

Wade, R. (1994). Teacher education students' views on class discussion: Implications for fostering critical reflection. *Teaching and Teacher Education, 10*(2), 231–243.

Weaver, R., & Qi, J. (2005). Classroom organization and participation: College students' perceptions. *The Journal of Higher Education, 76*(5), 570-601.

Weismer, M. (2007). Problem-based learning: Benefits and risks. *The Teaching Professor, 21*(2), p. 5.

Zlotkowski, E. (Ed.). (2001). *Successful service-learning programs: New models of excellence in higher education*. San Francisco, CA: Jossey-Bass.

7

Assessing Student Learning

> *Assessment efforts should not be concerned about valuing what can be measured but, instead, about measuring that which is valued.*
> —Banta, Lund, Black, & Oblander (1996)

Assessment is a term used in many contexts within discussions related to contemporary practices in higher education. Practices surrounding assessment allow for faculty to gauge how well their students have mastered certain aspects of course content in a variety of ways. Some readers might find the link between teaching and assessment to be tenuous, at best, although we would argue that they're actually very closely related educational practices. If teaching reflects the practices faculty apply to assist students in coming to a new understanding about a particular set of topics or ideas, then assessment measures the success of not only students in learning the material, but the suitability and sustainability of our teaching methods and curriculum, as well (Fook & Sidhu, 2010).

As we've laid out in previous chapters, teaching is a process that should encourage active involvement on the part of students in order to engage them fully in the learning process. Yet, this sort of teaching isn't necessarily compatible with the traditional forms of assessment that we might remember from our own experiences as students. If we engage students in constructing their learning, is it acceptable to give them a multiple-choice test to measure their learning? Or, can the process of learning itself be assessed as a measure of student achievement? These questions are just a few that support the notion that assessment is a tricky endeavor. Indeed, it can be unwieldy and complex, necessitating much thought and reflection by course instructors if it is to be approached correctly. That said, the bottom line for us is that evidence-based assessment should be the outcome of EBE. In this chapter, we outline some of the primary categories of assessment, explain their uses within a college-level classroom, and provide examples of how each can be applied within the study of speech-language pathology and audiology.

Overview of Assessment

Assessment can be a product or a process. As faculty, you can *create* an assessment to be used to measure student learning, or you can *engage* in assessment to gather data for a particular purpose (e.g., measuring learning, improving teaching). It is the latter idea of assessment for which we have an affinity. Although the actual construction of an assessment (e.g., creation of an assessment tool) is important, we believe that the process inherent in conducting and implementing an assessment is most critical to effectively understanding outcomes for both students and teachers. Faculty who truly understand the process of assessment recognize the need to engage in differing types of assessment practices depending on the information they hope to collect. Further, they comprehend the idea that learning (and teaching for that matter) can be evaluated in a layered fashion, wherein multiple types of assessment can be implemented simultaneously as part of a well-conceived assessment plan.

Assessment Approaches

Knowing what assessment is constitutes the easy part of the evaluation process. The most difficult decisions lie in determining what should be assessed and how the assessment process itself should proceed. Fortunately, faculty have several choices to draw from in forming a process for assessment, which mirrors their needs within a given context.

Summative Assessment: Assessment of Learning

Summative assessment is considered to be a comprehensive form of assessment wherein students are evaluated to determine their level of mastery across a given body of information at a given point in time. Summative assessments typically take the form of an objective test administered to students at the end of a unit, chapter, or term within a semester. For this reason, summative assessments can be referred to as *assessments of learning* (Black, Harrison, Lee, Marshall, & Wiliam, 2003) as they typically contribute to course grades based on specific criteria or standards (Lim & Rodger, 2010). Examples of summative assessment practices commonly used by CSD faculty include the following:

- Multiple-choice test questions
- True/false test questions
- Essay test questions
- Comprehensive exams for program completion
- Comprehensive programmatic exams such as the PRAXIS for professional licensure and/or certification

The biggest concern with the use of summative assessments is that they often fail to take learner diversity into account. Students' needs, interests, and ways of learning are different from one student to the next, and the application of a one-size-fits-all approach to assessment isn't the most valid method of honoring these student differences (Fook & Sidhu, 2010). Boud (2000) has urged faculty to move toward a more sustainable form of assessing students' performance in order to drive learning beyond an individual test to long-term learning, which can be applied in multiple contexts over time. Researchers agree that while summative assessments can provide a standardized snapshot of achievement across students, assessment should allow for learning to have "life beyond the end of [a] course" (Fook & Sidhu, 2010, p. 154).

Formative Assessment: Assessment for Learning

Formative assessment is defined as all activities which, when undertaken by teachers and/or students, can provide information that helps to modify teaching and learning practices (Black & William, 1998). Some consider formative assessment to be a measure of learning with understanding as opposed to simple memorization of information, as it encourages ongoing monitoring of acquired skills in order to facilitate learning (Harlen & James, 1997). Formative assessment typically occurs for smaller pieces of information at one time than is seen with summative information. Thus, formative assessment is seen as an assessment of one concept or idea within a course, rather than a reflection of learning on a larger scale. Although formative assessments can be graded, the purpose of formative assessment is to provide information to improve student learning, not data for use in computing course grades (Angelo & Cross, 1993). Figure 7–1 demonstrates formative assessment as a cyclical process, one in which the process of formative assessment is part of a continuous loop involving feedback, student engagement, and data gathering.

For these reasons, formative assessment could be conceptualized as *assessment for learning* (Black et al., 2003) as data obtained through formative assessment is used to identify gaps in student learning or to drive instructional change. Leahy, Lyon, Thompson, and Wiliam (2005, p. 23) specify that "teachers using assessment *for* learning continually look for ways in which they can generate evidence about student learning, and they use this evidence to adapt their instruction to better meet their students' learning needs." Table 7–1 outlines the characteristics of strongly designed formative assessments.

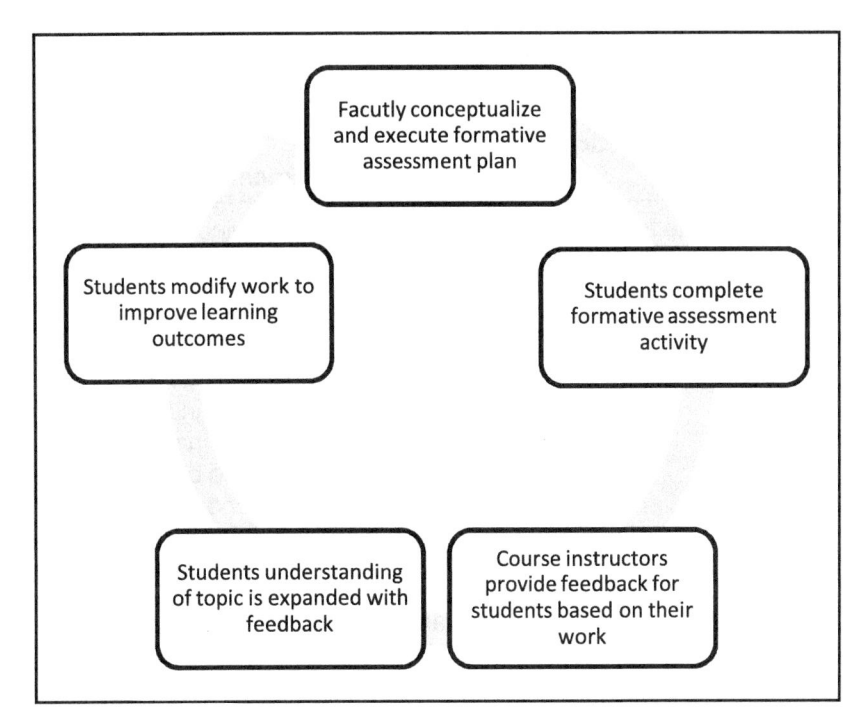

Figure 7-1. Cyclical nature of formative assessment. Based on Cauley and McMillan (2009).

The cycle shows: Facutly conceptualize and execute formative assessment plan → Students complete formative assessment activity → Course instructors provide feedback for students based on their work → Students understanding of topic is expanded with feedback → Students modify work to improve learning outcomes → (back to start).

Compared with summative assessments, formative assessments typically yield more favorable outcomes in student learning due to the engaged nature of the learning activity itself (Craddock & Mathias, 2009). Further, formative assessment has been described as effective in identifying gaps in course curriculum, driving instructional change, and scaffolding student learning (Fook & Sidhu, 2010). Examples of activities that might be used as part of a planned formative assessment in a CSD course include the following:

- Participation in structured class discussions about a controversial treatment protocol
- Completion of group work to gain mastery of a particular course topic
- Use of journaling or portfolios to provide and elicit faculty/ student feedback or reflection

Table 7–1. Qualities of Effective Formative Assessment Practices

High Quality Assessment Practices Should:	Rationale/Importance
Directly relate to learning objectives and other curricular activities	There should be an obvious connection between course content and any assessment to ensure student learning, engagement, and participation.
Be purposeful and goal directed	Many formative assessments are brief measures of understanding. To maximize benefit of formative assessment, there should be clear guidance for students and course instructors with regard to procedures and expectations.
Be both relevant and engaging	As many formative assessments are worth few points in relation to larger projects/exams, students will need to see the "buy in" for the work they're doing.
Provide timely feedback for students	Since the purpose of formative assessment is to identify and correct errors, feedback is a critical part of the process. Feedback must be provided to ensure that change (either from students or from instructors) can be facilitated.
Be part of an ongoing process of assessment	Formative assessment can and should happen more than one time a semester. Continued opportunities for course instructors to view student performance and provide appropriate feedback leads to increased student learning across the semester.

Source: Adapted from Paul University (n.d.).

- Peer review of written work to assist in editing, expanding, and comprehension of new material
- Use of collaborative group testing, in which quizzes initially are completed by each individual student, then collaboratively in groups
- Allowing students to teach other students in the class, as it has been suggested that students learn best when they have to teach the information to others (Michael & Modell, 2003)

Authentic Assessment: Assessment for Practical Learning

Authentic assessment takes the foundation of formative assessment and expands its boundaries to include an emphasis on real-world application as a component of any assessment activity. By this description, authentic assessment could be viewed as a subset of either formative assessment, depending on its application within a particular academic context. And, although the differences between summative and authentic assessment might be clear to teachers, the difference between formative and authentic assessments might be less so. Overall, the main difference between formative and authentic assessment lies in that real-world application. Formative assessments don't have to have that aspect built into their design; when they do, the assessment is considered to be authentic in nature. The idea behind authentic assessment is to provide opportunities for students to demonstrate knowledge in a manner that allows for easier generalization beyond the boundaries of the academic setting. Thus, what is learned can be revisited in a more realistic (nonclassroom) setting at some point in the future. We view authentic assessment as the perfect complement to a clinical field of study such as CSD, as faculty must work to prepare students for eventual clinical careers. For these reasons, we view authentic assessment as *assessment for practical learning* as data collected in this style of evaluation leads to an idea of how students will apply learning in practical settings outside of the classroom environment.

Examples of activities that could be used as part of an authentic assessment plan within a CSD course include the following:

- Use of case studies to problem solve assessment or treatment issues centered on a particular topic or disorder
- Completion of a language sample collection/transcription/analysis project to assess student ability to assess morphosyntax
- Development of a hearing conservation program for drum corps musicians to assess students' skills/understanding of primary prevention practices

Summative, Formative, and Authentic Assessment in Practice

It is important to view these varied options for assessment in context to understand their possible uses. We would urge faculty to understand that it is possible (and even preferable!) to use more than one form of assessment within a given class. Research supports this notion and indicates that any theory about different types of assessment should include some reference to other types of assessment to better depict the cyclical process inherent within valuable assessment experiences (Sebatane, 1998). Faculty can navigate from one type of assessment back to another as is appropriate for a given course. The question then becomes, what sort of assessment should be used at a given point within a course? Figure 7–2 presents our model for a combined assessment approach for faculty and students, understanding that the combination of assessment approaches likely leads to the best triangulation of student assessment data.

To address the question of what type of assessment to use in different contexts, we would suggest that the type of assessment faculty use should depend on the purpose of the assessment itself. Why? We assess students at different points in a semester for very different reasons and our assessment practices should reflect that difference in design and principle. Logically, then, faculty must be able to identify the reasons they might choose to assess student learning. Kellough & Kellough (1999) identified six specific purposes for assessment:

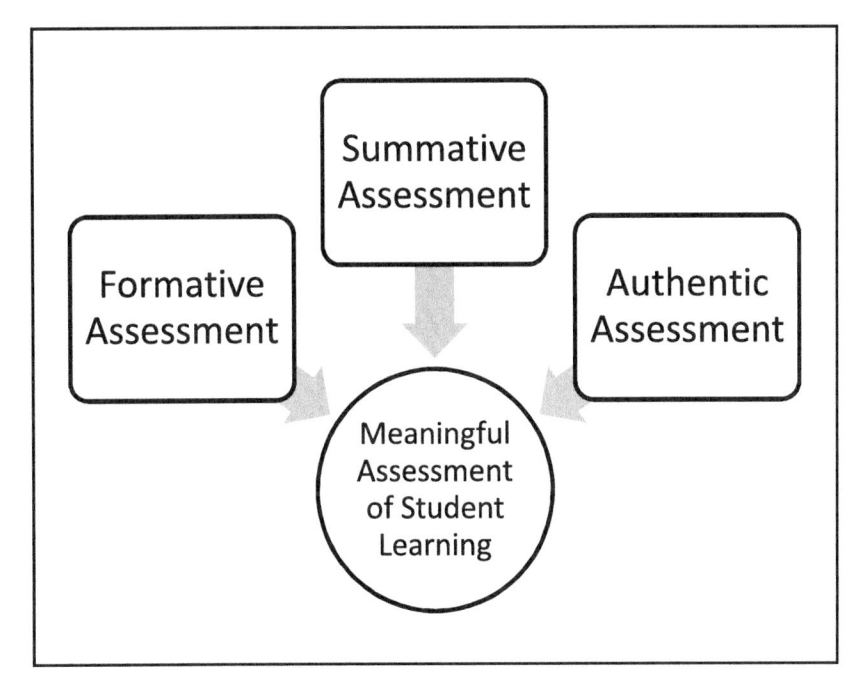

Figure 7–2. Model for classroom assessment.

1. To assess student learning
2. To identify student strengths and weaknesses
3. To assess the effectiveness of a particular pedagogical strategy
4. To assess the effectiveness of various curricular programs
5. To assess or improve teacher effectiveness
6. To provide data to assist in decision-making (pp. 418–419)

Could you use any type of assessment to achieve these six assessment purposes individually? Not likely. However, it would be possible to address each of the previously listed purposes for assessment using a combination of assessment approaches over the course of a given semester. Figure 7–3 details how a course instructor could use a variety of assessment techniques to measure students' understanding of grammatical morphemes. Additionally, Vignette 7–1 provides an example of how mixed assessment methods could be integrated into a CSD course.

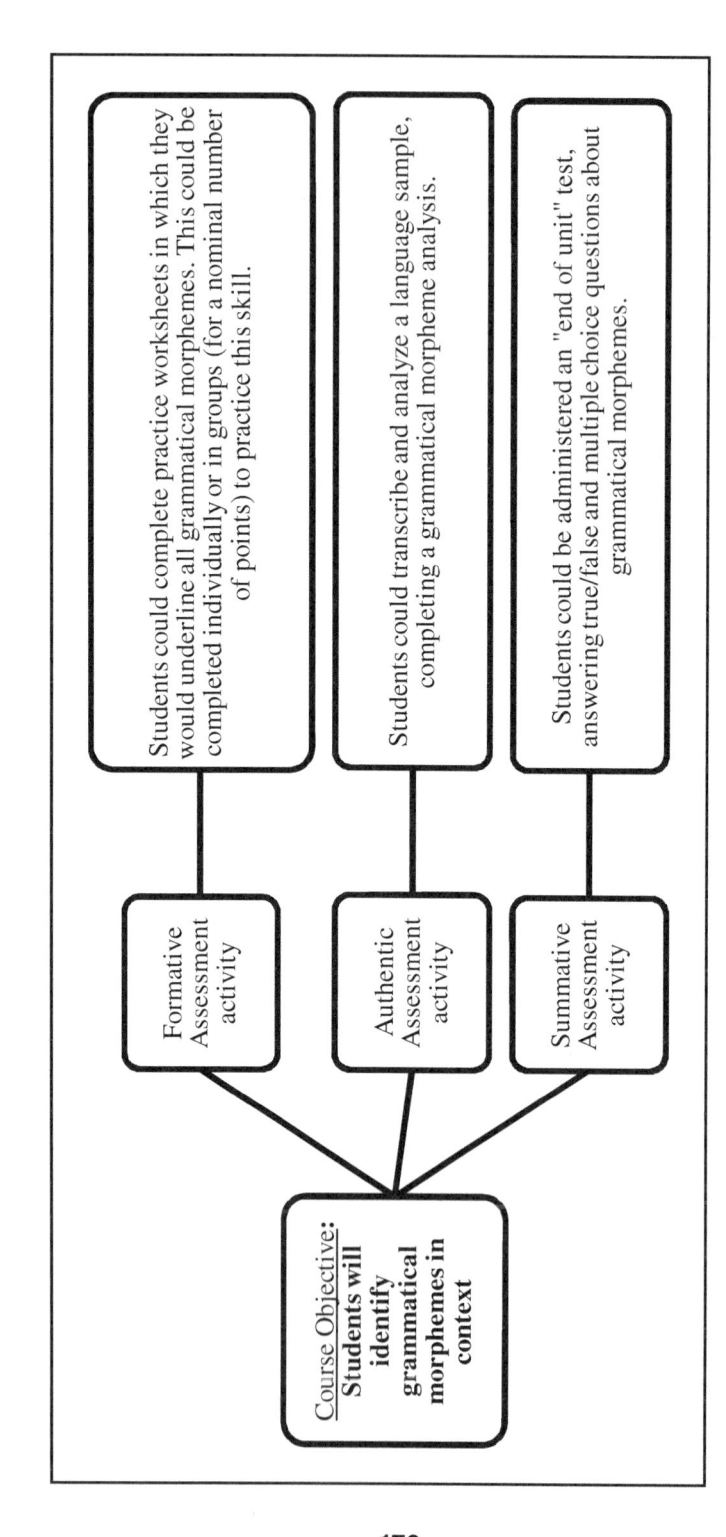

```
┌─────────────────────┐         ┌──────────────────────────────────────┐
│ Formative           │─────────│ Students could complete practice     │
│ Assessment          │         │ worksheets in which they would       │
│ activity            │         │ underline all grammatical morphemes. │
└─────────────────────┘         │ This could be completed individually │
                                │ or in groups (for a nominal number   │
                                │ of points) to practice this skill.   │
                                └──────────────────────────────────────┘

┌─────────────────────┐         ┌──────────────────────────────────────┐
│ Authentic           │─────────│ Students could transcribe and        │
│ Assessment          │         │ analyze a language sample,           │
│ activity            │         │ completing a grammatical morpheme    │
│                     │         │ analysis.                            │
└─────────────────────┘         └──────────────────────────────────────┘

┌─────────────────────┐         ┌──────────────────────────────────────┐
│ Summative           │─────────│ Students could be administered an    │
│ Assessment          │         │ "end of unit" test, answering        │
│ activity            │         │ true/false and multiple choice       │
│                     │         │ questions about grammatical          │
│                     │         │ morphemes.                           │
└─────────────────────┘         └──────────────────────────────────────┘

┌─────────────────────┐
│ Course Objective:   │
│ Students will       │
│ identify            │
│ grammatical         │
│ morphemes in        │
│ context             │
└─────────────────────┘
```

Figure 7–3. Application of varied assessment types in context.

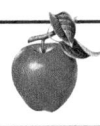

> **Vignette 7–1.** Example of Mixed Assessment Types in One Course
>
> Imagine you teach a graduate stuttering course. As your semester begins, you notice that your students have varied levels of understanding of stuttering. You realize that you need to gather information to allow you to make decisions about how to proceed with your course content to ensure that all students are starting with the chance to succeed. To accomplish this, you create a formative assessment in which, after viewing videotaped speech samples, students complete an individual class assignment detailing their impressions of the severity of stuttering and identifying secondary characteristics associated with each sample. This is not a graded assignment, but one that is valuable, nonetheless. You read and interpret student answers, providing written feedback to support or refute student perceptions. Your feedback provides resources for students to access to further their understanding of stuttering, as well. You make revisions to your syllabus for the semester, as you had presumed that students were coming to your course with knowledge they didn't actually possess. Thus, your assessment data was able to provide support for student learning while simultaneously informing teaching.
>
> As the semester unfolds, you determine a need to assess your students' strengths and weaknesses in designing treatment plans for children who stutter. You design an authentic assessment to allow students to partner with practicing speech-language pathologists to observe and assist in a fluency assessment, making treatment recommendations part of this experience, as well. Students present cases in "grand rounds" fashion to the class and present various treatment ideas, options, and recommendations. Using an analytic rubric (Table 7–2), grades are given to students, which reflect the effort, accuracy, and professionalism inherent within the final product.
>
> Finally, as the semester ends, you desire to measure your students' learning over the course of the semester. You decide the best way to do that is to create a summative assessment which will test students' knowledge in a broad manner. You design an objective test with multiple-choice, short answer, and essay questions. Grades reflect student accuracy in answering questions.

Table 7-2. Analytic Rubric for Vignette Example

Component	0 points	2 points	7 points	10 points
Define at least two fluency treatment approaches	Major flaws in your description of the treatment approaches, the materials, instrumentation, equipment, and/or the methodology; not appropriate for client.	Significant flaws in your description of the treatment approaches, the materials, instrumentation, equipment, and/or the methodology; not particularly appropriate for client.	Some minor flaws in your description of the treatment approaches, the materials, instrumentation, equipment, and/or the methodology; treatment is generally appropriate for client.	Generally appropriate for the client. Excellent presentation of your description of the treatment approaches, the materials, instrumentation, equipment, and/or the methodology. Appropriate approaches for client.
Discussion of the evidence for treatment	Evidence for the treatment not provided, not sufficient in depth, or not related to treatment approach.	Significant flaws in your discussion of the evidence for the treatment approaches, or the evidence is limited or lacks depth.	Some minor flaws in your discussion of evidence for the treatment provided.	Excellent discussion of treatment and exceptional evidence provided for the treatment.

Component	0 points	2 points	7 points	10 points
Demonstrate two possible therapy exercises	Treatment approach(es) not demonstrated; treatment is only described.	Significant errors in the treatment approach demonstration. Demonstrates some approaches, but not all.	Some minor errors in the treatment approach demonstration. Demonstrates most approaches, but not all.	Creative and exceptional demonstration of all of the treatment approaches.
Grammar, mechanics, etc., for handouts/presentation	Numerous, distracting errors in grammar, spelling, or punctuation. Poorly organized presentation and/or handout. Handout and/or presentation is not professional. Information is not presented at an appropriate rate. Reading directly from notes	Frequent distracting errors in grammar, spelling or punctuation. Frequent errors in the organization of the handout. Aspects of the handout and/or presentation are distracting. Frequent errors in the rate that the information is presented. Reading too much.	Some nondistracting errors in grammar, spelling, or punctuation. Some minor errors in the organization of the handout, or other aspects of the handout, and/or presentation are distracting. Minor errors in the rate that the information is presented. Only occasionally reads from notes	All aspects of the handout and presentation are excellent. Statements are well constructed, and handout is professional in its appearance. Information is presented at an appropriate rate. Does not read from notes. Tells the audience about the information

Tools for Assessment

Fortunately for faculty, several practices can be applied to the pursuit of evidence-based assessment. These are flexible tools that allow for a great deal of customization by faculty to address course-specific needs or other situational constraints. Two specific assessment tools that we feel are particularly successful in driving high-quality educational practices are rubrics and classroom assessment practices. Both are described in detail in the following sections.

Rubrics

Rubrics have been used widely in higher education as a tool to facilitate assessment for learning. Although used predominantly for grading work involving writing, rubrics have been used successfully to score group work, projects, and oral presentations (Moskal, 2000). Rubrics are used by faculty to communicate expectations for a given assignment or project by outlining criteria for its completion (Reddy & Andrade, 2010). Typically, as part of the process of articulating requirements, rubrics also provide students a sense of how levels of task mastery will be judged in a range from poor to excellent. Rubrics can be used as part of a formative of authentic assessment process (Popham, 1997) and have been demonstrated to not only quantify performance, but provide feedback for students detailing ways to improve performance (Moskal, 2000). Research suggests that rubrics increase the validity of formative assessment because they provide the following benefits (Andrade, 2000):

- Rubrics are easy to use and explain.
- Rubrics help to define and clarify teachers' expectations.
- Rubrics provide richer feedback for students relative to their areas of strength and weakness.
- Rubrics support learning by encouraging learner self-assessment.
- Rubrics support increases in the quality and skill evidenced in students' written work.
- Rubrics encourage good thinking by encouraging students to make judgments, organize work better, and drive higher level thinking.

Types of Rubrics

Rubrics are uniform across uses in that they are meant to assist in assessing student performance. That said, differences exist in how rubrics are designed, specific to how assignments and projects are graded with their use. Two predominant types of rubrics are used by faculty: analytic and holistic. Analytic rubrics are those that identify and assess separate components of a given project (Moskal, 2000). These rubrics allow for student work to be deconstructed into major components, each of which is assigned a grade. An overall grade is calculated by factoring in grades earned on each major component. In contrast, holistic rubrics are characterized by all project criteria being listed within a single descriptive scale, so work is not judged by the quality of its constituent parts, but as one finished product (Moskal, 2000). Course instructors choosing to develop rubrics to evaluate students' work must understand the difference between these rubric types and should consider carefully which might be more appropriate to the task at hand.

Tables 7–3 and 7–4 provide examples of the different types of rubrics that could be applied to the same potential class project to assess student work. Assuming students were tasked with reviewing peer-reviewed journal articles to establish an evidence base for a particular treatment approach, either the analytic rubric (Table 7–3) or holistic rubric (Table 7–4) could be used to provide students with feedback for their efforts and to assign a grade in a systematic manner.

Standards and Criteria for Rubric Use

Although course instructors can design and customize rubrics to fit many different pedagogical needs across a wide spectrum of classes and clinical experiences, certain components of rubrics should remain static across exemplars. Reddy and Andrade (2010) suggest that any rubric designed for use as an educational assessment should contain three distinct features:

1. Evaluation Criteria: Evaluation criteria are factors that help determine the quality of a student's work. These criteria can be weighted equally or differently depending on the style of rubric used and the relative importance of each criterion.

Table 7-3. Example of Analytic Rubric for Article Review Assignment

Content Area	Evaluation Criteria		
	2 pts.	1 pt.	0 pts.
Rationale for study/research questions	Clearly summarized rationale for study. Reader understands why study was conducted and what questions research was conducted to answer.	Brief overview of study's rationale provided, though it might be lacking in sufficient detail for readers to fully understand either the rationale and/or research questions for the study.	Rationale for study/research questions not included in review.
Study hypothesis not reported in review.	Hypothesis of study is clearly stated.	Hypothesis is reported in a vague manner, which is difficult to understand	Study hypothesis not reported in review.
Description of study methodology	Clear explanation of how study was carried out provided with sufficient accompanying detail.	Methods section of study is summarized in an unclear manner, with reader unable to understand how study was carried out.	Methods section not reported in review.

Evaluation Criteria

Content Area	2 pts.	1 pt.	0 pts.
Overview of findings	Findings are summarized precisely and accurately with sufficient detail to contextualize data reported.	Findings reported in vague manner with few details. Some inaccuracies in interpreting study findings might be evident.	Findings not reported in review.
Explanation of clinical application(s) for findings	Review provides clear idea of how findings related to direct clinical services. These clinical applications are clearly defined and explained.	Review provides a limited view of how findings relate to clinical service provision. Explanations are lacking in specificity and clarity.	Clinical application(s) of findings not discussed in review.
Grammar/spelling	Paper is free from grammatical/spelling errors.	Paper has few grammatical/ spelling errors.	Paper has more than three grammatical/ spelling errors.

Table 7–4. Example of Holistic Rubric for Article Review Assignment

Skill Rating	Points Earned	Content Description
Proficient	5 points	Review of article provides detailed, relevant information related to the rationale for the study, study hypothesis, methods used to test hypothesis, findings, and clinical application(s) of findings. Review is cohesive with few, if any, errors or omissions.
Satisfactory	3 points	Review of article provides satisfactory overview of rationale for the study, study hypothesis, methods used to test hypothesis, findings, and clinical application(s) of findings, although review is lacking in specific detail and might have minor errors in interpretation of the study being reviewed.
Limited/ Incomplete	1 point	Review of article is limited in scope and lacks thorough explanation of the study's rationale, hypothesis, methods, findings, and/or clinical application(s) of findings. Review is inaccurate and/or incomplete in scope.

Ideally, analytic rubrics should contain 3–5 evaluative criteria, with each identified criterion reflecting a key attribute or skill you wish students to master through the process of completing their work (Popham, 1997).

2. Quality Definitions: Quality definitions represent detailed descriptions of what students must achieve in order to be judged as proficient with a skill being assessed. These quality definitions are set on a continuum, representing low, medium, and high performance at a minimum. Quality definitions are consistently used in both analytic and holistic rubric designs.

3. Scoring Strategy: Scoring strategies are designed to quantify student performance in achieving proficiency on the evaluation criteria listed on a rubric. Scoring strategies generally invoke the use of a scale to represent different grades for varying levels of performance, relative to the quality definitions which are part of the rubric design.

Understanding that some components should remain similar across rubrics, we acknowledge that course instructors have a great deal of leeway in the actual design process when creating a rubric for use. To help ground faculty as they undertake the design of a new rubric, we've gathered recommendations from relevant research to facilitate this process. Brookhart (1999) and Andrade (2000) have outlined steps for faculty to follow in the design of assessment rubrics. Using these as the foundation for understanding quality rubric design, we would offer the following suggestions for faculty seeking to design a valid and reliable rubric:

1. Prior to beginning work on your rubric, review rubrics used by others for ideas and methods. Determine whether you will design an analytic or holistic rubric to meet your assessment needs.
2. Identify the content that needs to be included in students' work in order for proficiency with a given topic to be demonstrated. These content areas are your evaluation criteria. Combine and edit these criteria to ensure they aren't too lengthy or complex (information contained within rubrics should be easy to understand and follow). As information identified in this step will represent what you deem to represent proficiency with a given skill, these criteria will become the top levels of performance on the rubric. Note that if you choose to use a holistic rubric, you will identify only one evaluation criterion for use.
3. A continuum for performance needs to be created, with a range of achievement from low to high being represented. It has been recommended that varying performance levels be defined with exemplars (e.g., project displays five examples of primary prevention practices) rather than statements of judgment (e.g., "good" use of examples to illustrate point).

4. Create a draft of your idealized rubric and revise it, as needed. We would recommend that prior to initial use of any rubric, it is reviewed or pilot tested. Course instructors can ask a peer to edit/review new rubrics. Additionally, students can evaluate the rubric to ensure ease of comprehension of all aspects of the rubric by those who will be using it.

Classroom Assessment Techniques

Classroom Assessment Techniques (CATs) are used in conjunction with formative assessment practices as tools to collect data to support student learning (Angelo & Cross, 1993). CATs themselves aren't intended to replace other sorts of assessments but were established to structure simple exercises faculty could utilize in their classrooms to easily gather and analyze. CATs have proven efficacy as a pedagogical tool to assess student learning and drive higher-order thinking skill development (Davidson, 2009).

Angelo and Cross (1993) have described 45 different CATs that can be used to achieve the following purposes:

1. Assessing prior knowledge and understanding of course material
2. Assessing critical thinking
3. Assessing creative thinking
4. Assessing problem solving
5. Assessing application and performance
6. Assessing student awareness of their learning and performance
7. Assessing learner reactions to teachers, teaching, and classroom work

Beyond the purposes for the use of CATs in higher education, the benefits of using CATs have been detailed by several researchers. These benefits, stratified for both teachers and learners are summarized in Table 7–5.

We have culled through these CATs and have selected several for further examination here, as they can be immediately (and eas-

Table 7–5. Benefits of Classroom Learning Techniques

Benefits of CAT Use for Students	Benefits of CAT Use for Faculty
• Help students take responsibility and ownership for their own learning. • Give students a voice in their education, making them actively involved in their learning experiences. • Receive feedback that allows for modifications to learning/studying practices.	• Provide simultaneous short-term feedback regarding student learning and your own teaching, allowing for changes to teaching before the end of the term/semester. • Provide useful data related to student achievement in (often) a more efficient format than traditional assessments allow. • Support relationship building with students as they take an active role in shaping their academic experiences • Engage in a formative assessment process which evolves over time, leading to a never static, always evolving process for teaching.

Sources: Based on Angelo and Cross (1993) and Davis (1993).

ily) applied as a formative assessment tool for most CSD classes, regardless of course size, format, or level. Five specific CATs are described briefly in the following sections and are followed by Table 7–6, which provides examples of how these CATs could be applied within a CSD classroom setting.

Minute Paper

The Minute Paper is one of the most widely applied CATs in contemporary university teaching (Angelo & Cross, 1993). To facilitate the use of this CAT, faculty ask one of the two following questions in the final minutes of a class period: (1) *what was the most important thing you learned during this class?* and/or (2) *what important question do you have about this topic that remains unanswered at this point?* Students take a minute or two and formulate a written response to the question posed. Faculty review this information to gauge how well students are learning the material being presented in class on a given day and then make changes as indicated to improve students' understanding of important concepts.

Muddiest Point

The Muddiest Point CAT is meant to provide feedback to faculty related to what aspects of a particular concept remain unclear to students following a class meeting. Course instructors facilitate the use of this CAT by asking students to briefly respond to a question similar to *what was the muddiest (least clear) point in class for you today?* Students respond to this question in writing for faculty to review and respond to in subsequent class meetings or via other class communication.

One Sentence Summary

The One Sentence Summary "enables teachers to find out how concisely, completely and creatively students can summarize a large amount of information on a given topic" (Angelo & Cross, 1993, p. 183). To use this CAT, course instructors ask students to draft a one sentence summary to represent a course topic or reading. This CAT allows faculty to view how well students are able to synthesize learned information in their own words, with the understanding that students who don't completely comprehend a topic will struggle to summarize it accurately.

Applications Cards

Applications Cards present the opportunity for faculty to encourage student generalization of new information to more real-life situations. To facilitate this CAT, course instructors disseminate an index card to each student following discussion of an important principle, theory, or procedure in class (Angelo & Cross, 1993). Students are asked to write at least one real-world application for what they've just learned to share with peers and/or the course instructor. This CAT allows faculty to assess how well their students can apply and synthesize new information in a useful manner.

Everyday Ethical Dilemmas

Within the context of this CAT, faculty present students with short, direct case studies, which contain some sort of dilemma that calls into question the ethics of the situation described. Students are asked to identify (verbally or in writing) the ethical dilemma and present ways in which the dilemma might be handled or solved. This CAT allows faculty to track students' ability to take and defend differing perspectives, make ethical decisions, and revise clinical practice to improve outcomes.

Chapters 4, 5, 6, and 7 in our book was designed to make faculty critically consider the practices we engage in on a day-to-day basis as teachers as we strive to be evidence-based educators. We have highlighted what we view as the most salient aspects of class design, classroom communication, student engagement, and assessment of learning for course instructors and would encourage reflection on these practices as readers work toward making changes to their teaching in the future. Looking forward, we have much to learn in speech-language pathology and audiology about how we teach and how our students learn. Thus, we find the charge for engaging in SOTL research to be of great importance for academicians in CSD. To this end, the third and final section of our book is dedicated to helping faculty either begin or enhance work on their own SOTL research agendas.

Table 7-6. Application of CATs in CSD Classrooms

	Examples of Possible CAT Applications:	Modifications in Teaching Driven by CATs:
Minute Paper	After a class meeting in which working with diverse cultures in clinical settings was discussed, the course instructor asks students to write a brief paragraph detailing the most important professional practice issue they can identify as a result of class discussions/readings/etc.	Faculty member can read over students' Minute Papers and discern whether discrepancies exist in what the intended learning goal was for class and what the actual learning outcome was, and subsequently arrange to review information in future class meetings to clarify and extend on student learning.
Muddiest Point	Understanding that teaching the intricacies of cranial nerve functions can lead to some uncertainty among students, a course instructor teaching a clinical neurology course could ask that following the presentation and discussion of cranial nerves in class, students take a minute or two to detail any confusion they have related to cranial nerves and their role in supporting communication.	Faculty member can read students' responses and readily identify information that needs to be revisited in the next class session to ensure students have grasped the concepts and ideas critical to understanding the innervations and function of various cranial nerves. Topics requiring further clarification can be discussed prior to the introduction of new material to ensure students have the best possible chance to build on a solid understanding of course material.

	Examples of Possible CAT Applications:	Modifications in Teaching Driven by CATs:
One Sentence Summary	A course instructor working to facilitate a discussion related to evidence-based clinical practice might begin class one day by asking students to each provide a one sentence summary that defines and describes evidence-based practice. These one-sentence summaries could be shared in small or large groups and could serve as the basis for class discussion.	By listening to the one-sentences summaries as they're shared among students, the course instructor immediately can estimate students' level of understanding of evidence-based practice and can structure discussion, lecture, and other learning activities to complement students' needs.
Applications Cards	After reviewing stages of language development in a graduate language disorders class, a course instructor could disseminate index cards to students and ask them to conceptualize a diagnostic observation, which would allow for assessment of language development in an academic or social context.	The course instructor could review these application cards, provide individualized feedback for students, and ascertain students' ability to take information and use it in a manner consistent with higher-level thinking (analysis and synthesis). The course instructor could provide scaffolding to students struggling to make the leap from theory to application, thus driving student learning.
Everyday Ethical Dilemmas	A faculty member teaching an amplification course for graduate audiology students might present a case study wherein hearing aids are being distributed online with no in-person clinical service provision. As part of a class discussion, students could be asked to identify ethical issues arising in this situation and brainstorm ways to work around situations in a positive, professional manner.	Throughout this process, the faculty member facilitating this discussion can ascertain the level of understanding her students have related to ASHA's Code of Ethics and can garner an idea of how her students apply their knowledge to solve real clinical problems. The faculty member can intervene to present evidence-based suggestions where warranted to enhance student understanding of the issues being discussed.

References

Andrade, H. (2000). Using rubrics to promote thinking and learning. *Educational Leadership, 57*(5), 13–18.

Angelo, T., & Cross, K. (1993). *Classroom assessment techniques: A handbook for college teachers* (2nd ed.). San Francisco, CA: Jossey-Bass.

Arter, J., & McTighe, J. (2001). *Scoring rubrics in the classroom: Using performance criteria for assessing and improving student performance.* Thousand Oaks, CA: Corwin Press.

Black, P., Harrison, C., Lee, C., Marshall, B., & Wiliam, D. (2003). *Assessment for learning: Putting it into practice.* Berkshire, UK: McGraw-Hill.

Black, P., & Wiliam, D. (1998). Assessment and classroom learning. *Assessment in Education, 5*(1), 7–74.

Boud, D. (2000). Sustainable assessment: Rethinking assessment for the learning society. *Studies in Continuing Education, 22*(2), 151–167.

Brookhart, S. (1999). The art and science of classroom assessment: The missing part of pedagogy. *ASHE-ERIC Higher Education Report, 27*(1). Washington, DC: The George Washington University.

Cauley, K., & McMillan, J. (2009). Formative assessment techniques to support student motivation and achievement. *Clearing House, 83*(1), 1–6.

Craddock, D., & Mathias, H. (2009). Assessment options in higher education. *Assessment and Evaluation in Higher Education, 34*, 127–140.

Davidson, J. (2009). Preceptor use of classroom assessment techniques to stimulate higher-order thinking in the clinical setting. *Journal of Continuing Education in Nursing, 40*(3), 139–143.

Davis, B. (1993). *Tools for teaching.* San Francisco, CA: Jossey-Bass.

Fook, C., & Sidhu, G. (2010). Authentic assessment and pedagogical strategies in higher education. *Journal of Social Sciences, 6*(2), 153–161.

Harlen, W., & James, M. (1997). Assessment and learning: Differences and relationships between formative and summative assessment. *Assessment in Education, 4*, 365–379.

Kealey, E. (2010). Assessment and evaluation in social work education: Formative and summative approaches. *Journal of Teaching in Social Work, 30*, 64–74.

Kellough, R., & Kellough, N. (1999). *Secondary school teaching: A guide to methods and resources; planning for competence.* Upper Saddle River, NJ: Prentice Hill.

Leahy, S., Lyon, C., Thompson, M., & Wiliam, D. (2005). Classroom assessment: Minute by minute, day by day. *Educational Leadership, 63*(3), 19–24.

Lim, S., & Rodger, S. (2010). The use of interactive formative assessments with first-year occupational therapy students. *International Journal of Therapy and Rehabilitation, 17*(11), 576–586.

Michael, J., & Modell, H. (2003). Active learning in secondary and college classrooms: A working model for helping the learner to learn. Marwah, NJ: Erlbaum.

Moskal, B. (2000). Scoring rubrics: What, when and how? *Practical Assessment, Research & Evaluation, 7*(3). Retrieved from http://www.pareonline.net/getvn.asp?v=7&n=3

Park University. (n.d.). *Formative assessment in the classroom.* Retrieved from http://www.park.edu/cetl2/quicktips/formative.html

Popham, W. (1997). What's wrong—and what's right—with rubrics. *Educational Leadership, 55*(2), 72–75.

Rao, P., Collins, H., & DiCarlo, S. (2002). Collaborative testing enhances student learning. *Advances in Physiological Education, 26*(1), 37–41.

Reddy, Y., & Andrade, H. (2010). A review of rubric use in higher education. *Assessment & Evaluation in Higher Education, 35*(4), 435–448.

Sebatane, E. (1998). Cited in Brookhart, S. (2001). Successful students' formative and summative uses of assessment information. *Assessment in Education, 8*(2), 153–169.

8

Moving Forward Toward SOTL

> *Put simply, future faculty deserve the opportunity to be prepared for success.*
> —Seidel & Montgomery (1996, p. 2)

Why We Need to Support Good, Scholarly Teaching and SOTL

University Support

In the first two sections of this text, we have introduced you to basic concepts related to the scholarship of teaching and learning (SOTL), distinguished between various levels of teaching proficiency, and shared a variety of evidence-based educational (EBE) strategies for teaching and learning success. In this section, we want to discuss ideas that will help move doctoral students and faculty alike forward, toward maximizing their teaching effectiveness and, if interested, toward taking the first steps of engaging in SOTL.

We can begin by examining why universities, on a larger scale, should support SOTL. It is important to note that even at postsecondary institutions where research is dominant, there is still some acknowledgement of the value of teaching or education in the institution's mission statement. However, a disconnect may exist between a university's stated mission of providing a quality, meaningful, transformative learning experience and how they achieve that. In order for faculty to provide the best learning experience possible, they must be supported by the institution itself. The institution needs to look at the barriers and supports that they create in order for faculty to fulfill this portion of their mission. Fink notes, "Effective instructional development is linked to and depends on effective organizational development" (2003, p. 199). According to Fink's model, in order for a college to be effective in educating its students, colleges must identify what good educational outcomes are expected, then align its educational programs with these goals, and create "organizational structures, policies and procedures" (p. 200) to support the programs and the faculty teaching.

Trying to gain a sense of the obstacles presented by organizational structures and policies that will be present at a new academic job is a challenge. When considering a job offer, new faculty often are most concerned with what will be required to achieve tenure at a given institution. This is understandable as tenure is an enormous hurtle that means the difference between staying someplace for as long as you desire and having to pick up and start all over again in a few years. Tenure also implies a level of competence to the broader academic community and may suggest, at some institutions, a higher degree of academic freedom both in and out of the classroom. Often information about tenure and promotion is found by talking to prospective colleagues or by reading union-related documents at a university where faculty are collectively bargained-for. However, how is the newly minted doctoral student to know whether the university has in place policies and procedures that will support her growth as a teacher as well as a researcher? This can be a large challenge as even prospective colleagues, depending on the value that they place on teaching, may not be able to answer succinctly.

One of us works at a university where the tag line is "Education First," but how would a potential new faculty member know whether it is meaningful or not? Here are a few items that you might want to investigate when considering a new job if you want to know whether the importance you place on teaching will be well matched by the college or university that is interviewing you. One of the most important organizational structures, noted in Chapter 1, and identified by Fink, is a "strong faculty development program" (2003, p. 203). In order to learn more about the support a university may offer, consider the following:

- Investigate what the campus' teaching and learning center offers.
- Look to see whether programs appear to offer content that will be challenging, helping you to expand your current knowledge about teaching.
- Examine the university's Web pages to see what types of teaching awards the institutions gives and the prizes associated with those awards. Large organizations tend to fund the initiatives that are truly important to them.

In addition to looking at the university Web pages for signs that teaching and learning is truly valued, talking to the people who work there can be very informative. These can be helpful to you, particularly if SOTL is critically important to you.

- Ask the people who work in the department and the administrators how good or scholarly teaching is supported.
- Inquire as to their perception of the required balance between good research and good teaching needed to be successful as a faculty member in that department.
- Look for SOTL programs across the campus and signs that other faculty are participating in SOTL.
- View faculty members' Web pages to see what activities are listed.
- Search for "scholarship of teaching and learning" in the university's search engine.
- Ask during the interview process whether SOTL research is accepted as part of a research agenda if you know that you will not be satisfied by taking a faculty position where SOTL is not valued.

No matter how you prioritize your teaching and research, knowing the university's stand on SOTL will help you make a more educated decision about taking a position. There is not a wrong type of institution for you to consider taking a faculty position in, but if you understand the match between their expectations and your priorities, you will likely have greater job satisfaction.

Doctoral Program Support

Closer to home in our own disciplines, we need to examine how we are preparing doctoral students for the role of teaching so that as new faculty, they are prepared to move toward scholarly teaching and SOTL, should they desire to do so. The primary role of postsecondary faculty was to provide education to students until the 1970s when the focus began shifting toward research and obtaining research funding (Orjada & Dachtyl, 2007). The shift in focus is particularly evident in research universities, often still referred to as "R1's" based on the former Carnegie Classification systems of the 1990s. Many of our doctoral programs in CSD are housed in the research intensive universities and focus most of their doctoral education on preparing strong researchers. The challenge is that not all graduates of these programs are likely to move into a faculty role in that same type of institution (Gardner, 2005). Although our field needs competent researchers in order to continue exploring our field and to add to the body of evidence based clinical practice, the reality is that the majority of faculty jobs are not at these types of research focused universities. According to the latest Carnegie Classification (2010), less than 10% of the colleges and universities in this country are considered research universities. If we are willing to accept that effective teaching is not simply a matter of standing in front of a group of students and lecturing at them, as the evidence in previous chapters has supported, then we need to consider how we prepare future faculty for their roles as researchers and as teachers at a variety of types of institutions where CSD educational programs are housed.

Data from the most recent Council of Academic Programs in Communication Sciences and Disorders Survey of Research Doctoral Students (2009) indicates that doctoral students in their first year of their programs at predominantly research universities were given opportunities for teaching, such as giving a lecture (50%), using technology in teaching (56%), and evaluating/grading assignments (41%). In contrast, only 17–31% of the first-year doctoral students had attended a formal workshop or course on teaching. This suggests a possible disparity between the teaching responsibilities given to first-year doctoral students and the commensurate preparations they are given in order to perform these duties. As students moved further into their doctoral education, they reported having more opportunities for learning about teaching and for more teaching responsibility. For students who had been in a doctoral program between 2 and 10 years, 91% reported giving lectures, 90% had used technology for teaching, and 84% had evaluated/graded assignments. Although their formal preparations for teaching increased, with 34–46% participating in a formal workshop or course on teaching, the numbers still call into question whether our professions are preparing new faculty adequately to teach—a responsibility that all faculty will share to some degree, independent of the type of institution in which they are employed.

Without formal education in university teaching, PhD students hold a limited view of instruction, despite having gained some experience in the classroom during their program. Harland & Plangger (2004) found that doctoral students viewed the act of teaching as being about knowledge dissemination or transfer, not about creating active, engaged learning environments. This perspective may have contributed to a lack of satisfaction with their teaching role. Further, because of the strong research focus of the doctoral programs, teaching activities were felt to be devalued within the program. However, past research has demonstrated that doctoral students who have more teaching knowledge and experience are seen as more desirable candidates for faculty positions (Orjada & Dachtyl, 2007). Doctoral students who have spent time and energy preparing to be effective teachers are less likely to be frustrated in their first year as faculty members because they will understand more of what is expected of them (Gardner, 2005) and will be better equipped to handle many of the challenges that we face when we are fully responsible for a course, such as managing grading challenges from students, misbehaviors such as plagiarism, and poor outcomes on assessments of learning (Orjada & Dachtyl, 2007). In addition, by being prepared to teach before taking on the faculty position, new faculty may be able to have more time and energy to focus on their research, writing, and development of their scholarly agenda in their early years as junior faculty (Orjada & Dachtyl, 2007).

If we are to prepare doctoral students for the role of teacher and faculty member, we must consider, as Fink suggested, more formal policies and procedures for supporting this learning. This call is not new, but is being repeated at this time and for our profession that is in desperate need of new, doctoral-prepared faculty (Gardner, 2005). A curriculum that includes teaching need not necessarily be in direct conflict with the research curriculum (Orjada & Dachtyl, 2007). Methods available for improving teaching effectiveness include formal coursework in teaching, having mentors specifically for teaching, expanded opportunities for teaching experience with the appropriate evaluation and feedback for teaching, and direct supervision of teaching, much as we provide graduate student clinicians (Gardner, 2005; Orjada & Dachtyl, 2007; Walstad & Becker, 2010). A teaching curriculum can be offered by a combination of people to be most effective. Portions can be offered by faculty developers who hold broad pedagogical knowledge, while faculty from within the discipline who are particularly well equipped to discuss pedagogical content knowledge can present other aspects of the program and can serve as mentors or role models (Walstad & Becker, 2010). In order to prepare doctoral students for learner-centered teaching and help them value their roles as teachers, we must place priority on their preparations during doctoral education. The next section identifies a number of these mechanisms that can be incorporated easily into doctoral education and new faculty support programs.

Mechanisms of Support for Professional Development Toward SOTL

Faculty Teaching and Learning Centers

In the first chapter of this book, the use of specific tools available from university teaching and learning centers (TLC) are noted for use by faculty desiring to grow along the continuum of professional development of teaching and learning. We mentioned several specific tools that commonly are available through centers that support teaching, including support for interpretation of teacher evaluations, collecting mid-semester feedback, and participating in learning communities. As noted in that chapter, it is possible to accomplish many positive outcomes with or without the use of a faculty consultant; however, we would like to highlight here the possible benefit to doctoral students and faculty of developing an ongoing relationship with the TLC as part of the forward movement toward scholarly teaching and SOTL as part of our professional development.

In her 2008 article, then Carnegie Foundation Vice President Pat Hutchings suggested that professional development should not be work that happens upon occasion, such as when faculty or doctoral students are facing a crisis in the classroom, but rather that the work needs to be reflective of ongoing efforts to improve teaching and learning. She referred to this process as one that is "sustained over time" (p. 1) in order to maximize the support a TLC can provide to any educator. A second principle that she identified for successful professional development through a TLC is that of collaboration. Instructors need, but often aren't afforded opportunities for, collaboration with each other and with faculty consultants. A TLC should not only offer the types of communities of practice outlined in Chapter 1, but also will work to structure opportunities for a variety of collaborations to occur for the benefit of all those engaged in the teaching process on a campus. Finally, Hutchings calls on professional development to focus, as we have here, on evidence about student learning. The effective TLC will provide educators with resources about EBE practices, as well as opportunities to explore, discuss, and study them. Highlighting this unique view of the work of the TLC can transform it from the "emergency room" for faculty in trouble to the teaching hospital model in which faculty attempt to identify problems, learn about them through research, and then feed the learning back into the educational system, creating a cycle by which educators at all different levels benefit from the insights of others (Bernstein & Ginsberg, 2009). As noted in Chapter 1, it is important to view the TLC as a place where discussions can be fostered in a safe, supportive environment without judgment as professionals work to improve their teaching.

Improving Teaching through Mentoring

Mentoring has been documented as an effective model of professional development, whereby the development is seen as a continuous process for improving "knowledge and skills required for effective professional practice" (Lopez-Real & Kwan, 2005, p. 16). Savage, Karp, and Logue (2004, p. 23) specifically suggests that mentoring can be used **for** "supporting a view of scholarship that includes the scholarship of teaching as well as applied research within a specific discipline." Mentoring is not a new model for ongoing professional development in academia, however it is changing shape and character. Mentoring at universities often is intended to help junior faculty learn about campus resources, department policies, and to promote general information sharing and problem solving (Savage, Karp, & Logue, 2004). Mentoring also can be used successfully to foster development in a particular area for doctoral students, such as pedagogy. Where the term mentor once implied a dyadic model of a senior, knowledgeable faculty member bringing along a junior, inexperienced colleague, new models are appearing that shift the focus from the mentor to the mentee and to a new process for mentoring (Darwin & Palmer, 2008; Savage et al., 2004). Rather than being paternalistic in nature (Darwin & Palmer, 2008), new mentoring relationships are described as being "learner centered" (Fischler & Zachary, 2009; Zachary, 2002) and "synergistic" (Goodwin, 2004) and no longer look like a one-to-one relationship of senior to junior. Modern mentoring is just as likely to include a group of people at varying levels of knowledge or achievement interacting in a "network" (Goodwin, 2004) or in a "circle" (Darwin & Palmer, 2008).

Synergistic mentoring is intended to be more reciprocal in nature than the dyadic models. One of the unique characteristics of this model is that both the mentor and the mentee are interested in pursuing a common interest or outcome (Goodwin, 2004). The learning is more mutual as both parties recognize that they each have the opportunity to learn from the other as they attempt some joint venture or learning. Sometimes referred to as "peer networking" rather than mentoring (Goodwin, 2004, p. 147), the relationship de-emphasizes the senior and junior roles and instead focuses on a shared support of growth. One of the functions that can be served by mentoring is to extend the doctoral student's knowledge and experiences in a particular area, such research or teaching. Pairing faculty and students who have a common interest allows the individuals to work together toward a joint conclusion or an outcome that both are invested in, such as the use of technology in undergraduate education. Connections around a common interest also facilitate both members of the mentoring relationship to bring some perspective or input to the process, further supporting the reciprocal nature of synergistic mentoring. It has been hypothesized that one reason for the success of this model is that adults tend to seek reciprocal relationships rather than one-sided, unidirectional relationships, creating a sense of equity in the learning and growing process (Goodwin, 2004). The synergistic mentoring model gives recognition to the strengths and knowledge that all parties bring to the process.

Another learner-centered model of mentoring is mentoring circles, which also may be referred to as group mentoring. Mentoring circles bring together a collection of people who are at a similar point in their educational or academic careers and will learn together and whose learning is facilitated by a mentor (Darwin & Palmer, 2009; McCormack & West, 2006). One of the most unique characteristics about mentoring circles is that they allow members of the group to mentor each other, along with the mentoring that they receive from the mentor-facilitator. The facilitator is supposed to keep the focus of the group's discussions on topic and productive, but may not have all of the answers to solve the issues that are being discussed in the circle. The facilitator, who is typically more senior or experienced, is able to provide resources and support for the group members, although the group dynamic recognizes the possibility of mentees learning from each other, as well as from the facilitating mentor.

The benefit of mentoring in higher education is well documented. Traditional mentoring in academic settings has been shown to improve career development and advancement, management of psychosocial issues related to academia, as well as increased self-confidence and personal satisfaction (Darwin & Palmer, 2009; McCormack & West, 2006; Savage, Karp & Logue, 2004). The additional benefits of mentoring circles over one-to-one mentoring relationships, include the opportunity to learn from multiple people, gain diverse perspectives, and the prospect of group members forming cohesive support networks that will likely extend beyond the formal mentoring process and time line (Darwin & Palmer, 2009; McCormack & West, 2006). This may help combat the sense of isolation that can occur for doctoral students and new faculty alike, and can aid in the forming of lasting, supportive relationships that can be instrumental as individuals advance within their careers. Additionally, mentoring circles have been shown to improve knowledge acquisition relative to the focus of the group, improve confidence, and change the culture of programs (Darwin & Palmer, 2009; McCormack & West, 2006).

Although the mentoring process has been demonstrated to be a valuable one for doctoral students and new faculty, it is not without significant challenges. Perhaps the most significant among the challenges to mentoring success is time (Darwin & Palmer, 2009; Savage, Karp & Logue, 2004). Faculty who are mentoring must make time in their busy schedules to reach out to those whom they are mentoring, schedule regular meetings, and plan for those meetings. Additional time challenges face the mentees as they struggle to include the mentoring meetings into their schedules of taking courses, new teaching assignments, developing a research agenda, and finding ways to work for others, either as doctoral student research assistants or in the role of faculty service. Another significant challenge to the success of a mentoring relationship is the personal connection between people (Darwin & Palmer, 2009; Fischler & Zachary, 2009; Savage, Karp & Logue, 2004; Zachary 2002). In one-to-one mentoring relationships, the parties may struggle with power differentials, mentors may lack a willingness to see the process as collaborative, and personalities may simply clash. Savage, Karp, and Logue (2004) note that doctoral students and new faculty may be apprehensive and mistrustful of mentors who are senior to them and may hold power over them in the form of grades or input for promotion. For mentoring groups or circles, compatibility of personalities across group members is essential if the group is to form a cohesive, supportive unit whose effects will be felt beyond the duration of the formal mentoring process (Darwin & Palmer, 2009). The final challenge that should be noted in mentoring relationships is the process of concluding them. Although some mentoring relationships will not have a finite ending date, many will, and Zachary (2002) suggests that the conclusion of the formal mentoring process or activities can bring anxiety for those in the relationship, particularly the mentees. She recommends that as the formal process comes to a close, an "exit strategy" (p. 36) be used that includes a conversation about what has been learned, how to move forward from that point, and if the relationship is to continue, how it will be redefined. It is important to note that while many of the mentoring relationships we engage in change over time, becoming more mutual, and possibly collegial in nature, some will end with the end of the specific mentoring activities. Planning for and discussing this eventuality may make this transition easier for all involved.

Mentors who are successful with new models are not dissimilar from successful mentors in the traditional model: They demonstrate interest and support of the mentee, are willing to share information, and are positive during the process (Goodwin, 2004). In addition, good mentors will understand that they are a resource for finding answers and giving guidance, rather than feeling that they should embody all of the knowledge that the mentee needs (Zachary, 2002). Zachary (2002) notes that effective mentors will involve learners, or mentees, in the planning of what will be learned and how, will help learners identify their own learning objectives for the mentoring process, and will adhere to the best practices of learner centered, adult learning strategies. Mentors also should be "reciprocal and collaborative" (p. 28). In other words, the process of being an effective mentor is very similar to that of being an effective teacher. Mentors who engage in successful mentoring relationships, independent of the structure of those relationships, often find that they benefit from the process just as the mentee does. In a study of mentors' perceptions of their own professional development, Lopez-Real and Kwan (2005) found that mentors learned more about their own professional practice as they were asked questions that caused them to reflect on their own teaching experiences. Mentors in this study also felt that they learned about new ideas and strategies from their mentees. This type of learning is not inconsistent with the professional satisfaction that we often hear from internship supervisors when they reflect on the benefit to them of supervising graduate student clinicians.

Peer Observation of Teaching as a Tool for Growth

In the first chapter, we mentioned that taking the opportunity to observe a highly thought of colleague teaching can be valuable to shaping our insights about what good teaching looks like. In this section, we are going to explore the idea of peer observation as a specific tool that is more complex than watching a good teacher teach once or twice. Here, we present the idea of peer observation as a means for ongoing professional development, one that is process-oriented rather than being an experience or practice that occurs in isolation of a context. Interestingly, the use of peer observations of teaching (POT) in higher education has been studied extensively in the United Kingdom and Australia as it is a practice that is widespread in their postsecondary educational institutions (Hammersley-Fletcher & Orsmond, 2004). The interest in POT originated from a government-led initiative that was attempting to improve the quality of UK higher education (Shortland, 2004). Also referred to as a peer review of teaching, it can be used for both summative assessment purposes, such as tenure and promotion decisions, but it is used primarily for formative assessment purposes. The University of Tasmania (The Higher Education Academy, 2009) notes that there are five main reasons that they use peer review of teaching, including:

1. Usefulness in creating a teaching portfolio
2. Ensures teaching quality
3. Expectation that it will lead to increased teaching effectiveness
4. Facilitates the exchange of knowledge regarding teaching and learning at the university.
5. Formally creates opportunities for discussions about teaching

Requiring POT across a university would be an example of a policy or procedure that would ensure increased support of teaching, as Fink calls for, noted previously.

Three possible models are available for peer-review processes. In the "evaluation model" senior staff completes the observing, much as we see in the evaluation process for tenure common on many of our campuses (Blackmore, 2005, p. 222). The "developmental model" (p. 222) is similar to what happens in this country if an instructor contacts their TLC and asks for a consultant or developer to come and watch their class, often in search of a solution to a particular problem. In this model, it is assumed that the observer has some specific expertise related to teaching and learning. Finally, the "peer review model" (p. 222), or POT model, which dominates the literature, is one in which teachers observe each other. There are no assumptions of seniority or higher levels of knowledge between participants.

With POT, doctoral students or new faculty work together in teams of their own choosing or can be assigned by someone else, such as an instructor or a department head. The teams can include three or four members, and the group members take turns observing each other, over the course of a year or multiple years (Blackmore, 2005; Shortland, 2004). The participants are playing both the role of observer and observee, over time, which aids in developing a mutual relationship, trust, and a focus so that issues related to teaching can be discussed credibly (Blackmore, 2005; Hammersley-Fletcher & Orsmond, 2005). Because of the reciprocal nature of these relationships, care must be given to how feedback is handled, and power struggles need to be avoided. Shortland (2010) suggests that it is not adequate to be sure that the individuals in a peer group are friends or are critical of each other. Rather, she advocates that peers should act as "critical friends" (p. 297), building on trust, empathy, and respect rather than emphasizing evaluation. When possible, mutual selection appears to be the most successful for choosing members of peer observation teams. Most importantly, the process is seen as being beneficial to all participants, not just the person being observed (Shortland, 2004).

Typically, four steps are outlined for engaging in POT, as shown in Figure 8–1. It again must be emphasized that in order for this process to be effective, the evaluative nature of the observation needs to be minimized, and a focus should be placed on constructive feedback and potential solutions to be beneficial to growth and development (Shortland, 2004; Shortland, 2010). Conversely, feedback that is too "self-congratulatory" is not helpful as it lacks honesty and accuracy, robbing the observee of the opportunity to learn and benefit from the POT process (Blackmore, 2005, p. 223)

Peer observation of teaching is intended to be a process that facilitates improved teaching by creating opportunities for reflection on teaching, addressing teachers' needs in terms of learning and growth about teaching, and stimulating discussion around best practices in higher education among colleagues. Reflection, which is felt to be a critical element for successful teachers, is fostered through the process of examining others' teaching and comparing it to their own teaching and knowledge (Hammersley-Fletcher & Orsmond, 2005). As the peer-review process fosters the reflections and peer relationships, it is thought that faculty will be open to innovations and changes to improve educational practice. Unlike individual workshops or one-time faculty consultations with a TLC, POT is a process that teachers engage in over an extended period of time.

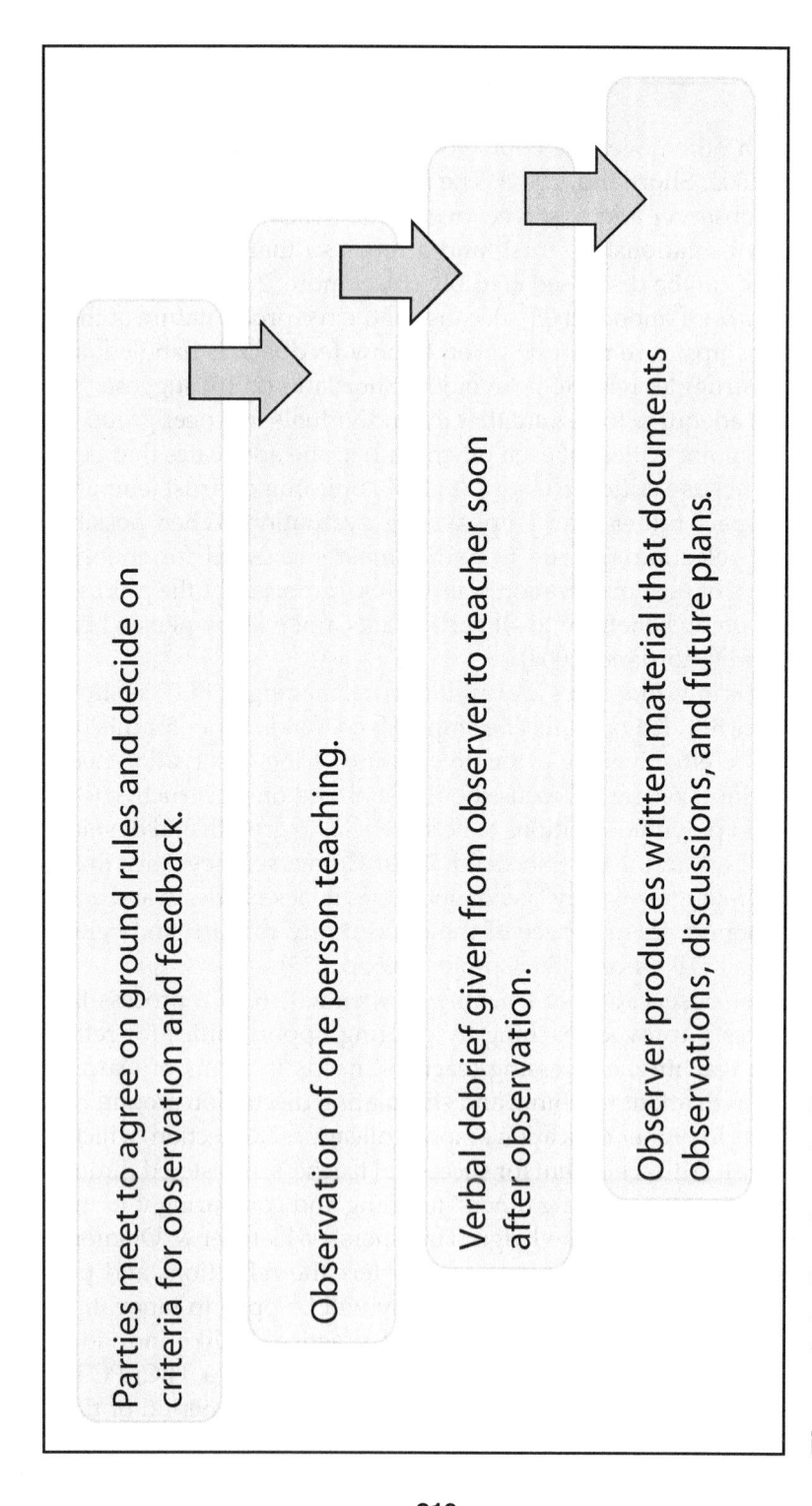

Parties meet to agree on ground rules and decide on criteria for observation and feedback. → Observation of one person teaching. → Verbal debrief given from observer to teacher soon after observation. → Observer produces written material that documents observations, discussions, and future plans.

Figure 8–1. Four Steps for Engaging in Peer Observation of Teaching. Based on Shortland, 2004, 2010.

The longer-term connections that develop from this process, much like mentoring, are felt to encourage a deeper level of learning that will be impactful/powerful in improving teaching (Shortland, 2004; Shortland, 2010).

Research on the effectiveness of POT has been generally positive, however there have been a few mixed results regarding the usefulness of peer observations for the purpose of professional development of higher education instructors. When meaningful dialogue, such as what takes place in the third step, is not a critical part of the peer-review process, participants are likely to not find it satisfying (Nixon, Vickerman, & Maynard, 2010). The voluntary nature of participating in POT was found to be important to some faculty (Atkinson & Bolt, 2010). Several studies have demonstrated that when a clear goal or focus of the observation is provided, teachers are more likely to find the process useful and valuable (Atkinson & Bolt, 2010; Hammersley-Fletcher & Orsmond, 2004). One study of POT targeted specifically teacher communication behaviors associated with immediacy (see Chapter 5) and found that by addressing a specific theme, faculty were able to make better use of the feedback to improve their teaching. A set of guidelines for best practices in the use of POT based on the current literature follows in Figure 8–2.

Teachers Researching Teaching: Action Research for SOTL

One of the questions that inevitably arises when we talk with colleagues about engaging in SOTL is the issue of the value or validity of conducting research in your own classroom. This leads us to conversations about how and where you might conduct SOTL research. It should be noted that SOTL research does not necessarily have to take place in your own classroom. Investigations about teaching and learning can be situated in a variety of contexts, including in programs that are comparable to your own, are very different from your own, or have some other set of characteristics in common, such as discipline, educational level, or educational model, that has little to do with the context in which you teach. The choice is yours to make

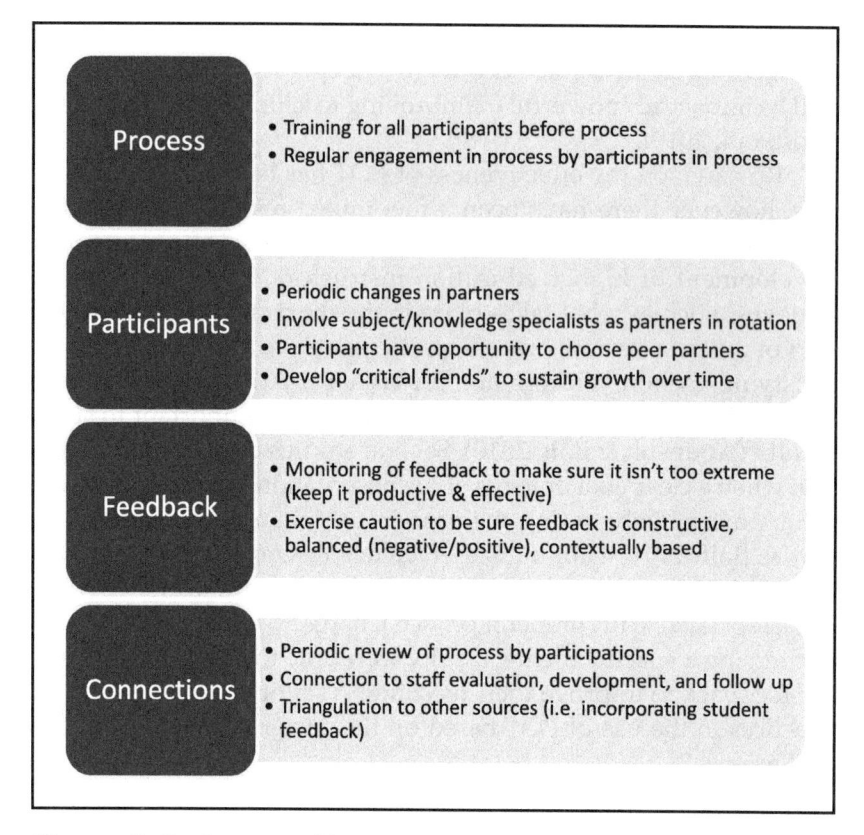

Process
- Training for all participants before process
- Regular engagement in process by participants in process

Participants
- Periodic changes in partners
- Involve subject/knowledge specialists as partners in rotation
- Participants have opportunity to choose peer partners
- Develop "critical friends" to sustain growth over time

Feedback
- Monitoring of feedback to make sure it isn't too extreme (keep it productive & effective)
- Exercise caution to be sure feedback is constructive, balanced (negative/positive), contextually based

Connections
- Periodic review of process by participations
- Connection to staff evaluation, development, and follow up
- Triangulation to other sources (i.e. incorporating student feedback)

Figure 8–2. Suggested Best Practice Guidelines for POT. Based on Blackmore, 2005, and Shortland, 2010.

and depends in large part upon your research questions and what you are hoping to accomplish through your research.

One common approach to engaging in SOTL research is to begin by looking at the questions that confront us about our teaching and learning in our own classrooms (McKinney, 2007). As referenced in Chapter 1, Bass (1999) highlights that problems in our teaching represent the same opportunity for investigation and learning as discipline-based problems do. Likely, all of us have had the experience of walking out of a classroom and thinking, "I wonder why that learning activity that seemed like such a great idea just flopped" or "Why did those students fail the assignment when I taught the information as well as I could?" Often these kinds of questions form the basis of good reflections on teaching and lead us to become more scholarly teachers as we seek out information in the literature about how to approach a learning activity or an assessment (Anderson, Herr, & Nihlen, 1996; Smith, 2008). In moving forward toward engaging in SOTL, these reflections must become more formalized inquiries.

There is a long-standing history of teachers engaging in *action research* to improve their understanding of educational process and student experiences (Esposito & Smith, 2006; Postholm, 2008). Eisner (1998) notes that qualitative inquiry in schools and classrooms has the dual benefit of teaching us about the learning that is happening in other classrooms as well as helping us understand what is happening in an individual classroom, such as our own. Without this understanding, he points out, we cannot educate others about how to be effective educators. Action research is rooted in the qualitative method. In the qualitative tradition, research often occurs in the midst of an on-going process, situated in a real-life context (Postholm, 2008). This work endeavors to make sense of the process being studied by understanding the perspectives of those who are participating in it. Sometimes, as in the case with action research taking place in a teacher's own classroom, the observer is a participant as well (Denzin & Lincoln, 2003). In action research, occasionally referred to as practitioner-research, the person conducting the study is also the person who is a practitioner, such as a faculty member. Research conducted with qualitative methods will not be replicable to the same degree as quantitative research is, however that does not make it less valuable for us as educators. As we read qualitative research that was well conducted and well written, the experiences of the researcher and the participants speak to the reader as an event or a perspective that has a ring of truth and familiarity to it. In other words, although the details of the specific context or participants may differ from our own experience, the story has a credibility and authenticity that we can relate to and learn from. In this sense, qualitative research can be considered "generalizable" (Denzin & Lincoln, 2003).

It is important to note that, as with all qualitative research, action research is "value-laden" (Postholm, 2008, p 146) in that there are strong connections between the person conducting the research and the research itself. This commonly is addressed by identifying, in the dissemination of the research, the teacher-researcher's position relative to the work that was done and the findings. This acceptance of a body of work that is influenced by the researcher's values is consistent with the post positivist perspective, although it often is rejected by positivist, hard science researchers (Denzin & Lincoln, 2003). As such, it may feel "squishy" to those used to the use of the experimental method of research (Smith, 2008, p. 266). Action research has been informing higher education to improve learning for a number of years (Esposito & Smith, 2006). One of the reasons it is thought to be effective is because the research is specific to the context in which the instructor is teaching. Teachers engaging in investigations of teaching and learning in their own classroom are improving their own teaching as well as looking beyond their classroom to inform us of best practices for other settings (Eisner, 1998; Paulsen, 2001). This type of research advances pedagogical content knowledge, as well as the scholarship of teaching.

One of the benefits of action research is its ability to provide insights into the *how* and *why* questions that we have about teaching and learning (Eisner, 1998; Paulsen 2001). Where quantitative data is able to demonstrate that students perform statistically better on a test when they were taught with Method X than when they were taught with Method Y, qualitative data gives insights into why Method X helped them have a better learning outcome than Method Y. It likely will shed light on the complex nature of teaching and learning by helping us understand it from the participants' perspectives. By using qualitative research methods, we are able to investigate many aspects of the teaching and learning dynamic. Additionally, the use of action research can be empowering to both the teacher and the students (Esposito & Smith, 2006). Teachers are likely to feel empowered as they learn more about the impact of their actions in the classroom, and as a result become more effective educators. Students are likely to feel empowered as they begin to understand that their opinions, perspectives, and outcomes can have an impact on their own education as they participate in action research. Vignette 8–1 highlights how one author uses action research in the classroom.

In order for questions that arise from our teaching to move forward to become SOTL, they must be formalized and held up to public scrutiny by our colleagues. As noted by Hutchings and Shulman (1999), SOTL work also must be made visible to our colleagues through public dissemination. This may take the form of presentations at academic conferences that peer-review submis-

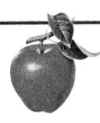

> **Vignette 8–1.** Types of Data I Collect
>
> I am a qualitative researcher simply because of the way my brain works. I have participated in quantitative research, but the questions that we were trying to answer never compelled me in the same way as the questions do when I am conducting qualitative research. In reflecting on what happens in my own classrooms, I tend to ask myself 'why' and 'how' questions, such as "how do the students feel about this?" and "why do some students learn better under certain conditions?" The data I collect reflects this. In many of my studies, I endeavor to understand more about the value of teaching or a communication approach from the students' perspectives by asking them. Most often, I engage student volunteers, sometimes in my own classes and sometimes in colleagues' classes, in individual, face-to-face, semi-structured interviews. Many of the questions that I ask the students seek to identify what aspects of the teaching-learning experience in a particular condition are salient to them. Most of my studies have investigated aspects of affective learning associated with effective teaching. For example, in answering a research question about classroom communication, I might ask students how a teacher's specific communication skills impact their perceptions of that teacher's effectiveness, or what they learn about that teacher from how he communicates with them. Through coding and thematic analysis of interview data, along with other data, such as interviewing the teacher, I am able to learn more about the students' perceptions of a teacher's communication in the classroom and how those perceptions impact their learning. In conducting SOTL investigations, I use qualitative methods because they not only answer my questions, but also because they help me understand the learner's perspective, which informs my understanding of teaching and learning in my own classroom. Insights into what our audience, the students, want and need to support their learning is a critical component for me in being an effective teacher.

sions or through publication in peer-reviewed journals. The work also should contribute to moving others' research forward to grow the body of literature that is available for EBE. Questions that examine the relationship between teaching and learning are often what we consider to be the hallmark of SOTL (Paulsen, 2001). Questions that are asked by our accrediting agencies, such as the Council of Academic Accreditation for ASHA and NCATE for those associated with professional education units, are often good places to begin. We might ask, for example, "What is the evidence that we use to determine that our students have learned what we expect them to learn?" or "What are students able to do after completing a specific portion of learning (such as a unit or whole class)?" (Smith, 2008).

Guided by our own reflections, by accreditation processes, or by our own burning questions, we can collect a number of types of data and we can design our studies of teaching and learning in a number of ways. For some of us, examining two groups of students in two different sections of the same class receiving differing forms of instruction can create opportunities to make a comparison of the impact of the teaching method present in one and missing in the other, akin to having a control group. If you don't have two sections of one class, it may be possible to compare data from classes you have taught over time or compare outcomes to a section being taught by a colleague (Smith, 2008). Some faculty have divided students into two random groups and presented material or learning activities to half of the class for half of a session and then taught the other half during the second half of a session, in order to be able to identify the value of the method used. It should be noted that many times a control group is just not feasible. If a control group is not feasible, either because you cannot incorporate the use of the design into your class or because you don't feel that withholding of a teaching technique is in the students' best interest (see "Ethical Considerations and SOTL" later in this chapter), then it may be advisable to collect careful and thorough data that compares what you are expecting your students to learn (learning outcomes) with your teaching approach (Hutchings, 2003).

Performance on a specific assessment, such as an in-class examination, is one method of identifying a relationship between teaching and learning that is comfortable to many faculty and provides us with a great deal of information about EBE. Alternative methods of assessing cognitive learning are available as well. Numerous studies of cognitive learning have collected data that assesses perceived student "learning loss," which involves asking students to rate the difference between how much they learned in a class and how much they think they would have learned with the ideal instructor

(King & Witt, 2009). Perceptions of affective learning can be valuable to understanding the teaching and learning dynamics as well. Numerous validated scales exist for identifying aspects of students' motivation, for example (Christophel, 1990). If you have a preferred method of conducting research within your specific disciplinary area, it might be most feasible to begin with collecting data in that way (McKinney, 2007). If you are used to using surveys to measure your clients' satisfaction with two different brands of hearing aids, for example, then using satisfaction surveys may be an easy place to start with your collection of student data. This is one way of easing into SOTL that can reduce stress as you begin a new realm of research.

In addition to collecting data about student cognitive and affective learning outcomes, we can ask students to tell us what is happening for them as they learn. Through qualitative data collection, we can gather data that asks students how they felt during a particular learning experience, what concerns they had about a method of teaching, or how a teaching structure supported their learning. In his seminal work looking at the difference between how history faculty and history students think, Wineburg (1991) began using a "think-aloud" technique that presents the study participant with a complex problem that needs to be solved and asks them to think aloud as they work their way through the solution to the problem. Wineburg noted that this form of data collection focuses on the "intermediate process of cognition, not just outcomes" (p. 497) as it asks people to share what they are thinking, not just how they arrived at their conclusion or whether or not the conclusions are correct. Since this ground-breaking work was conducted in history, it has been replicated to great effect in countless disciplines.

Ethical Considerations and SOTL

Teacher versus Researcher

As noted previously, in the discussion of course design and action research, we must work through a number of ethical dilemmas in conducting SOTL. Some of these issues may be endemic to conducting research that includes humans, but for those of us who are engaged in action research in our own classrooms, we need to take some special consideration of what we are doing and why. We would be wise to remember, that much like physicians taking the Hippocratic oath that we should, as teachers "first, do no harm." Unfortunately, unlike physicians, we as teachers or faculty members have no such guiding code of ethics that we clearly all agree to and follow the ASHA Code of Ethics is principally oriented toward clinical practice. As a consequence, a great deal of gray area exists in the complicated decisions that we make as teachers, let alone as teachers endeavoring to engage in research in our classrooms (Burman & Kleinsasser, 2004). As we design our SOTL research, it is critical that we do not willingly or knowingly offer any group of students a substandard education. We cannot justify withholding that which we believe to be critical to their learning in order to make a good comparison between those who receive and those who do not receive a particular form of teaching. If we do not believe that an available method of teaching is effective, it cannot be used for a control group. As one professor put it, "The class is a class first and a research laboratory second; the students are students first and research subjects second" (Hutchings, 2003, p. 29). If you cannot wholeheartedly endorse a method of teaching, it should not be used as part of a study.

Even in a thoughtfully designed study that we feel good about, unexpected developments can occur that can significantly challenge our ethics as teacher-researchers. When we are conducting a purely experimental design study and realize that Treatment A is not working, we are probably unlikely to withdraw Treatment A from the study, unless it is potentially harmful to the participant. The study likely will continue to its conclusion at which point the data will be analyzed to determine that indeed, Treatment A was less effective than Treatment B. However, if we as teachers are studying how well something is working in our classroom and we realize, mid-study and mid-semester, that it is not working at all, is it ethical to continue? We think it is not. Following the directive that students are students first, research participants second, we believe that we must halt or alter the study in order to preserve the opportunity for learning and minimize the negative impact upon the students. It would be unethical to continue the study, knowing that our students are not learning what they need to learn from us in order to become competent clinicians. Vignette 8–2 describes the experience of attempting to collect a set of data and accidentally learning something you did not anticipate.

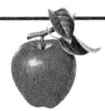

> **Vignette 8–2.** When My SOTL Study Went Off the Rails
>
> A couple of years ago I was conducting a study to learn about how undergraduate students felt about learning in a hybrid electronic class format. I designed an SOTL study that I planned to run in an undergraduate, 200-level course that I had been teaching for almost six years in a traditional format. After reading about hybrid course design in the literature, I created a hybrid format version of the course, applied for and received IRB approval, and set out to explain the study on the first day of class.
>
> As the traditional face-to-face portion and the hybrid online portion of the class progressed, it was clear that the students were making great connections between new content and their own lives. Through threaded discussions online and the dialogue in class, I had evidence that they were grasping the "big picture" concepts in this introductory-level class and were enthusiastic in their learning. I was thrilled that the level of energy, discussion, and connection appeared stronger than ever in this new hybrid format class. However, my euphoria quickly ended when I started realizing that the students' scores on the biweekly quizzes were much lower than was typical compared to past scores in the traditional format.
>
> As I discussed the apparent disconnect between an apparently eager group of learners and their poor quiz scores with a teaching and learning center SOTL group in which I was participating, I described the students' ability to wholeheartedly embrace what I referred to as the "big picture" concepts in light of their failure to learn the small details that were asked of them on the quiz. During this discussion, I realized that in revising my course to conform to the hybrid format, I had not anticipated the shift in focus that might occur from small details to overarching issues. Thus, I had not modified my assessments adequately to capture the students' learning.
>
> This new realization, arrived at in the middle of the semester, wasn't actually going to derail my study completely, as I wasn't collecting data about the degree of cognitive learning that the students

Vignette 8–2. *continued*

experienced, but rather focused on their attitudes toward the hybrid format. I was concerned, however, that they would be feeling frustrated about their low quiz scores and that this frustration would be reflected in the data that I was trying to gather regarding the format of the class. After mulling over the situation for several days, I decided to share my thinking with them and have an honest and open discussion with them about the connection between learning activities, learning outcomes, and assessments. As future clinicians and educators, all of these students would be faced with a problem of this sort somewhere in their futures. As I planned for the discussion, I wrote myself many notes, I outlined how I intended to approach the conversation with them, and when it was over, I wrote copious notes about how the students responded and what I learned from their responses.

It turned out that my students were more than receptive to this discussion. Initially, it was quiet, and then one of the more vocal students raised her hand and said "I think it is really cool that you are willing to talk about what is best for us with US!" That opened the floodgates, and a stimulating dialogue ensued. The students were empowered by my willingness to share my concern with them and ask for their input. We worked together to come to a mutually agreeable solution regarding the assessment, and the class ended on a positive note.

I felt that I had done the right thing, the ethical thing, all without necessarily sacrificing my SOTL study. But what the heck did I do with all of those notes I had made myself during the decision to have what my former Dean, Dr. Vernon Polite, might have called a "courageous conversation?" I knew that I had a reasonable study out from the data I had formally collected, but I felt like I was sitting on a goldmine of insight in these notes. As part of that TLC-SOTL support group in which I was participating, I was supposed to publish a chapter based on the SOTL research I was engaging in that term. I decided that rather than publish the results of the study, which were later published in Division 10's *Perspectives: Issues in Higher Education*, I would publish a reflective chapter that would share what I learned through making SOTL classroom community property, as Shulman refers to pedagogy brought out into the public light and made open for discussion. The chapter became a wisdom of practice piece that was gratifying to write and to get feedback on. I learned almost as much from the process that occurred in the middle of the study as I did from the study data. It was an invaluable experience for me as a teacher.

If you find yourself in this circumstance, do not fear that all is lost and you have wasted your time. If you recall from Chapter 2, in SOTL, unlike in much of our discipline-based research, there are opportunities for us to write reports based on the wisdom of practice. You may be able to write a personal account of change or a recommended practice report based on what you have learned in the process. You may be able to salvage your study with a new direction or new element added. Remember that this is typically not true of experimental design and that while your methods may change out of necessity, you have not necessarily lost the opportunity to learn about the relationship between teaching and learning in your classroom. In fact, you may learn more than you set out to learn. One helpful guideline to consider should you find yourself in this predicament is to keep careful notes about what is occurring, why you feel it is happening, and what you are doing to respond to the challenge. You might keep track of conversations you have with your students in and out of the classroom to record their view on the teaching-learning events with their permission. This can possibly become incorporated into your methods description and/or your conclusions, should your data be salvageable. If it is not, then your notes and reflections may become material for an excellent reflective piece that shares the wisdom of practice to guide others. In Vignette 8–3, one of the authors describes how she used unexpected information that came from data collection.

Institutional Review Board and SOTL Research

While the profession of teaching does not have one unifying code of ethics that we all agree to follow, researchers in this country must follow a very clear set of guidelines if the research includes any people. We must be aware of and adhere to a number of laws in conducting research with our students. The first is federal policy that appeared in the mid 1970s and sets forth guidelines regarding the rights of participants in research, such as the right to make decisions regarding their participation and the right to have their identity protected. Federal law regarding research with humans also protects participants by requiring researchers to provide them with informed consent, which lays out their rights as participants.

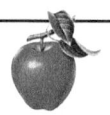

> **Vignette 8–3.** Moving into SOTL
>
> Approximately 5 years ago, I switched my pedagogical approach within all of my upper-level courses. I teach at an undergraduate-only program at a small liberal arts college. At the time that I made this change, I was the only full-time faculty member in the communication disorders program; therefore, I typically had the students in 5–6 different courses over the course of their 4 years, which meant they learned my teaching style and knew what to expect. I made the decision to spend part of my sabbatical examining various pedagogical approaches and decided to redesign my courses to utilize problem-based learning (PBL). In addition to redesigning my courses to incorporate PBL, I also decided to examine students' perceptions of their learning; therefore, I developed a survey to examine the students' perception of this new approach to learning. Specifically, the survey asked students about their perceptions regarding their learning, amount of work involved in the course, the use of PBLs, and development of a variety of skills (i.e., critical thinking, communication, research skills, etc.).
>
> The first semester that I incorporated PBL into my courses, I started the first class by explaining the changes and discussing what PBL was. The first PBL was an example that we worked on in class and that did not require any outside research in order to solve the problem. I then set off to have the students complete four PBLs during the remainder of the semester. The students met the learning outcomes for the course, performed well on the exams, and seemed more engaged with the course material both in and out of the classroom. In addition, their grades in the class were comparable to previous times that I had taught the course. I felt that this had been a successful pedagogical change. At the end of the semester, I invited the students to complete the survey regarding their perceptions. All of the students chose to complete the survey, and the results were not what I had expected. They understood the learning objectives for the activities, liked the active learning component to the PBLs, saw how the PBLs created an opportunity for them to apply class content to practical situations, learned to synthesize information, developed critical thinking skills and research skills, and improved communication; however, their comments were extremely negative. The comments included

statements such as "the PBLs did not help me learn," "PBLs are very stressful," "I found trying to learn in the PBLs were uncomfortable," "I feel like I learn better when the information is fed to me from the professor," among others.

I was discouraged. They were learning what I wanted them to learn, and they recognized the knowledge and skills that they were developing, but they were not seeing the value of the pedagogical approach. The students did not like the change. Being a bit stubborn, I did not want to give up on using PBLs in my classroom. After spending much of my summer reflecting and talking to colleagues about the student feedback, I decided that I needed to tweak the use of PBLs in my classroom. The one error that I made was that I did not clearly communicate with the students about my expectations and the roles that each of us would now have in the classroom. I decided that I needed to redesigned my syllabus to include what I called "Link Course Objectives, Activities, and Assessment," which provided the students with a rationale for what they were doing and how it related to the entire picture for the class. A few years later, I learned that this idea was very similar to what Fink (2003) discussed with regards to creating significant learning experiences (discussed in Chapter 4). In addition to redesigning my syllabi, I also decreased the number of PBLs in the course and made sure that I was helping the students to see the connections between the PBL task and the learning outcomes. Furthermore, I made sure that I explained my role in the PBL process.

The next semester things improved. The students were meeting the learning outcomes, and their comments regarding PBL were much more positive. Now that I have been using PBLs for many years and continuing to survey students about their perceptions, I have found that there are still those few students who just want to know what will be on the test, and so their comments tend to be more on the negative side, but these students are few and far between. In the end, I am glad that I made this pedagogical change. My classroom is an active learning classroom, and my students are engaged with the course content both inside and outside of the classroom. In order to complete the loop of SOTL, I have continued to not only collect data regarding the use of PBL and the students' perceptions to this approach, but to disseminate these findings at conferences and in publications.

Commonly, this document also lays out for the participant the expectations of potential harm and benefit that will come from their participation in this study. The age of consent for students is 18, based on federal law. For university researchers, this means that if you are including students who are younger than 18 in your study, you must get the consent of a parent or legal guardian for minor college students to participate. Along with the federal guidelines regarding research with people, we need to be mindful that other federal laws have an impact on us in university settings. For example, the Family Educational Rights and Privacy Act (FERPA) regulates the sharing of student information and the safeguard of student privacy and applies to students in most educational settings, from elementary school through doctoral programs (Burman & Kleinsasser, 2004).

Federal law regarding research involving people typically is monitored by a university's Institutional Review Board for use of human subjects, often referred to as IRB. It is the responsibility of the IRB to make sure that all members of a university community adhere to the laws that govern this research prior to the implementation of the study. For most IRBs, the process of reviewing proposals for discipline-based research is fairly straightforward. However, as the lines blur between teacher and researcher for SOTL, there may be confusion as to what is appropriate and acceptable practice (Burman & Kleinsasser, 2004; McKinney, 2007). Part of the confusion comes from the fact that within the Federal guidelines for research with human subjects, stipulates a number of categories of research that are "exempt" from IRB review. Several of the categories of research that are considered exempt apply to SOTL researchers, including (Burman & Kleinsasser, 2004, 67):

1. Research involving normal educational practices
2. Research using data from educational tests

This includes investigations of the "effectiveness of or the comparison among instructional techniques, curricula, or classroom management methods" (Hutchings, 2003, p. 30). One of the challenges is that at most institutions, the IRB actually will complete the review to determine whether the study qualifies for exempt status. Those unfamiliar with SOTL work may question why an instructor would collect data in her own classroom.

One of the reasons for the possible challenge of this research is the nature of the informed consent that must be completed by our students participating in SOTL studies. When research participants are provided with an informed consent, it not only spells out their rights, the potential benefits and harm that may arise from their participation, it provides them with the opportunity to decline the opportunity to participate. IRBs may call into question how free students may feel to say no to a faculty member asking for their participation in a study he is conducting in the same class in which he is assigning grades (Burman & Kleinsasser, 2004; Hutchings, 2003; McKinney, 2007). Where a potential exists for the perceived power of the faculty member to be coercive over the students being invited to participate in a study, the potential also exists for an IRB to reject the study on the basis that they do not feel it is possible to protect the participants and gain real consent.

In order to smooth the way for this process, there are a number of possible solutions (Hutchings, 2003; McKinney, 2007). The first, and possibly one of the most effective for bringing about a wholesale change for your entire institution, is to work with members of the IRB to help them understand the nature and value of SOTL research. Other solutions include having another faculty member or graduate assistant collect the informed consent documents that the students complete at the beginning of the term or the project and withhold them from the instructor-researcher until after grading has been completed. Some researchers choose to treat the students as collaborators in the research process, rather than as subjects or participants. In doing so, they hope to shift the power differential that may be felt by the students, as well as provide them with the increased engagement with their own education (Burman & Kleinsasser, 2004; Hutchings, 2003). Including students as collaborators in your research has the benefit of making them feel empowered about their education process and may have the added benefit of increasing their interest in research through active engagement (see Chapter 6). This perspective is consistent with the views many qualitative researchers have of their study participants, providing them with the chance to review what is written about them, which samples of their evidence are included in the study, and what pseudonym that they would like to be identified by (Denzin & Lincoln, 2003). In this vain, if you are going to include samples of your students' work in your disseminated results, it is important to offer them the opportunity to have their work attributed to them. Students whose work is presented as an exemplar of outstanding thinking, for example, may be very pleased to have their name appear in your article. However, students whose work may appear as examples of limited learning may not be flattered by having their name included next to the work. It is critical that we make it clear to students whose work is going to appear in a public forum that they retain control over that process (Hutchings, 2003; McKinney, 2007).

Hutchings (2003) notes that successful teacher-researchers make their intentions for research, including the nature and purpose of the study, clear to their students from the beginning. If we view the consent process not as simply asking the student to sign a document once, but instead see it as an ongoing process in which trust is developed and maintained over time throughout the research and education, then we may be better able to protect our students, consistent with the intent of federal law (Burman & Kleinsasser, 2004). After examining the potential ethical conflicts that SOTL researchers might face, Burman and Kleinsasser (2004, p. 69) created a list of principles that can be used to guide SOTL researchers in general and the use of student work in particular. Table 8–1 details these principles and possible ways to implement them. Vignette 8–4 looks at gaining IRB approval for a SOTL study using problem-based learning.

Dissemination of SOTL Work

As we have already discussed, SOTL work does not qualify as such unless it is publicly disseminated (Hutchings & Shulman, 1999; McKinney, 2007; Shulman, 2004). What public dissemination means can be a topic of discussion, depending on your setting and the criteria associated with that setting (see Chapter 9 for more discussion). It is commonly accepted in academia that dissemination that is public and subject to peer-review, as Shulman calls for, includes presentation at conferences where submissions are peer-reviewed and publication in juried journals. In deciding what format you would like to make your results public, you should consider the type of reward structure that your institution places on such efforts for the purpose of

Table 8-1. Principles Guiding the Use of Student Work in SOTL

1.	Identify as SOTL	Be sure that everyone involved, including graduate assistants, teaching assistants, and students, understands that this is a research project. Clarify your intentions openly through discussion.
2.	Plan your research	Before you begin your research and class, plan out all of the details about how your teaching, assessment, learning outcomes, and data collection will work for the course.
3.	Design informed consent process	Emphasize the notion that informed consent with our students is an ongoing process. Present regular opportunities for students to communicate with you, in and out of class, about how they are feeling about being part of the study.
4.	Seek external review	External review may take the form of approval from the IRB or from more informal sources, such as your department colleagues and peers whose opinion you trust.
5.	Inform students	Keep students knowledgeable about the research process throughout the term or during data collection so that they feel engaged in the process.
6.	Acknowledge student control	Let students know whether you intend to use their work and offer them options for how that work might be presented. Keep in mind that the work is theirs, and they should feel that they retain control about how it is presented in your study.
7.	Proceed carefully	Be cautious if you are trying to compare current work to the work of previous students if you did not obtain informed consent at that time.
8.	Consider involving students	Giving students more opportunities to be involved in your SOTL work, as collaborators, as peer-checkers, or in data analysis, increases likelihood of their feeling empowered and engaged in learning. It also may increase their interest in research.

continues

Table 8–1. *continued*

9. Share findings	Purposefully share what you're learning or have learned with your students in class. This again increases their sense of empowerment and provides them with closure as to what you did with their work. It also demystifies the SOTL research process, increasing the likelihood of other students' willingness to participate in similar studies in the future.

Source: Based on Burman and Kleinsasser, 2004, p. 69.

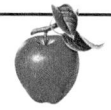

Vignette 8–4. Handling an IRB Issue

Much of my SOTL work revolves around the use of Problem-Based Learning (PBL) and student's perceptions regarding this approach to the teaching and learning of the course content. I approach this research by inviting students to complete various surveys regarding their knowledge and skill development within various courses. The students provide their consent when they agree to complete the survey. The only identifying information is their student identification number and the course number that they were enrolled in which PBL was utilized. As discussed earlier in the chapter, this type of SOTL research study means that the project falls into the exempt category for the IRB. It is exempt in this case because it is conducted in established or commonly accepted educational settings, involving normal educational practices, and the research involves the use of surveys. Even though it is exempt, I still had to get IRB approval in order to be able to share the findings beyond my own classroom.

The IRB approval process for exempt projects at my college is a quick and straightforward process that involves completing the appropriate IRB forms and writing a brief description of the research project that includes the research question(s), methodology, and the survey. Ideally, IRB approval should be sought prior to the course and project starting, but at the latest, it must be sought of all participants before presenting the findings outside of the department.

tenure and promotion. You also might consider the state of your work, how complete it is, and whether you are looking for an opportunity for feedback rather than being prepared to publish.

As you consider the value of the various forms of public dissemination for your SOTL work, you also should consider the within-discipline nature of your work in contrast to the opportunity to share your work in a setting that is more cross-disciplinary. In much of his writing, Shulman calls for SOTL work to be situated within the researcher's discipline (2004). He does so, in large part, because he recognized that in order for our SOTL work to gain the acceptance of our disciplinary colleagues, we must conduct research that is comparable to, or accepted by, those within our discipline. Those who judge us within our discipline will apply the same standards that they apply to our disciplinary research to determine its value. Additionally, he notes that professions each have their own signature pedagogy (Shulman, 2004) or a set of characteristics and expected outcomes that are held constant within a profession, across higher education settings. By having SOTL work reside within the discipline, there is the increased likelihood that our work will feed into and support our signature pedagogy. Work within a specific discipline holds the potential to inform the pedagogical content knowledge (PCK) that is unique to speech-language pathology and audiology.

Certainly, Shulman's points regarding the inclusion are well founded and have great merit. However, Weimer (2008) argues that the greater good of the academy would be better served if we were to position SOTL work in more broad contexts. She argues that by encouraging SOTL work to reside solely within the discipline, the need for duplication of efforts is increased as we are unlikely to search the SOTL publications of other professions in search of articles that will be useful to us. She notes that there is a certain level of redundancy in the type of work found in SOTL journals that are organized by discipline-based audiences. By not disseminating SOTL work in broader contexts, we do not have the opportunity to learn from each other. Although investigations about aspects of our teaching may be very unique to speech-language pathology or audiology, there is a great deal for us to learn from related fields that have similar learning structures. For example, SOTL work being conducted by a colleague in occupational therapy on the formation of professional identity of students during an internship experience has a great deal of potential to generalize to speech-language pathology. If an article resulting from this work is published in an occupational therapy journal, it will not be seen by faculty in our field and we won't be able to benefit from the work as we might if it were published in a more general SOTL context. Your decision to pursue dissemination within your discipline or across disciplines will depend on your personal preferences, your institution's criteria for acceptability, and the outlets that are available to you.

We have found that conference settings, particularly those that are on the slightly smaller scale of hundreds rather than thousands, are an ideal setting for the presentation of SOTL work that is relatively new and is perhaps not quite in its most finished form. At SOTL conferences, you are likely to find an audience that is not only interested in your ideas, your research, and your findings; you also are likely to find an audience that will give you feedback and reactions. Feedback of such nature, which in this setting tends toward positive and thought provoking, can be invaluable as you move your work toward its final stages and begin preparing for submission to a journal. A number of conference venues are peer-reviewed and focus on SOTL across a variety of disciplines. These conferences range in size and scope from more regional to international and are a wonderful opportunity for doctoral students and new faculty to become more acquainted with what colleagues across the academy are doing that may be related to your work or inspire your work. Conferences such as these also can be a useful support mechanism for people conducting SOTL work in the absence of colleagues on your own campus engaging in the same type of work or if your institution does not have its own teaching and learning center (TLC). For conference opportunities that focus on SOTL work, consult with your own TLC or use your favorite search engine to look on the Web for "scholarship of teaching and learning conferences."

If you desire to pursue a peer-reviewed publication of your SOTL work, you should consider a number of items. As noted previously, you will need to reflect on the acceptability of a publication that is not based in the discipline and your need for such publications for tenure and promotion. At the time of this writing, limited opportunities for publication exist within speech-language pathology and audiology for SOTL work. However, a number of broader journals are not discipline specific and seek to publish SOTL work. As with searching for conferences, consult your TLC or the Web for "scholarship of teaching and learning journals." If you decide to submit a manuscript to such a journal, a number of considerations are unique to cross-disciplinary journals that will help you be successful in having your manuscript accepted for publication.

As with all research, you need to ensure that there is a good fit between your research and the audience the journal you are considering (Maurer, 2011; McKinney, 2007). Moving outside of our own discipline means that some journals will be more appropriate than others for the publication of our work. For example, a faculty member who has researched issues of teaching and learning in an online classroom context might look to distance learning journals as well as SOTL journals for appropriate homes for her article. Ask yourself who might benefit from what you have learned and what journals are read by that audience. When you identify the journal you wish to submit to, research the journal online, looking to see what type of work they accept, such as quantitative work, qualitative work, and reflection pieces to be sure that your work is appropriate to this outlet. Carefully scrutinize the format details that they ask submitters to conform to as they may be different than the journals with which you have experience. Not following these submission guidelines may decrease your likelihood of acceptance (Maurer, 2011).

If you decide to submit your manuscript to a SOTL journal, you should follow a number of other guidelines. Remember that others reading your work will not be familiar with the jargon of CSD. You will need to minimize jargon and explain basic concepts in ways which you do not expect to do for a publication within the discipline (Tagg, 2011). Remember that many of the readers of a SOTL journal know little or nothing about speech-language pathology or audiology. Be sure that as you set up your research question in the first portion of your paper, you provide a context that helps the reader understand why the question is important and how the problem is gripping for those readers outside of your discipline (Bernstein, 2011). Consider the benefit of a broader perspective so that your audience can find the take-home lesson in your work, no matter what they teach. One effective way of doing this is by looking beyond CSD for your literature review and conceptual framework to connect your work to the broader body of research that is available (Tagg, 2011).

As you make the decision to move forward and engage in SOTL, you will have many choices and opportunities before you. Beginning with mechanisms that can improve your teaching also can increase your reflection upon it, such as through the mentoring route, or engaging in peer observation of teaching. This is often the first step toward identification of problems or questions that exist for you in regard to the teaching and learning process. After you have learned, reflected, and considered how to formalize your questions, you will be well on your way to engaging in SOTL. Remember that numerous sources of support are available for you on this journey, including teaching and learning centers, colleagues within the discipline at your own institution, across the country, and colleagues across disciplines.

References

Anderson, G. L., Herr, K., & Nihlen, A. S. (1996). What does practitioner research look like? *Teaching and Change, 3*(2), 173–206.

Atkinson, D. J., & Bolt, S. (2010). Using teacher observations to reflect upon and improve teaching practice in higher education. *Journal of Scholarship of Teaching and Learning, 10*(3), 1–19.

Bass, R. (1999). The scholarship of teaching: What's the problem? *Inventio: Creative Thinking About Learning and Teaching, 1*(1), 1–10.

Bernstein, J. L. (2011). Identifying high quality SoTL research: A perspective from a reviewer. *International journal for the Scholarship of Teaching and Learning, 5*(1). Retrieved from http://academics.georgiasouthern.edu/ijsotl/v5n1.html

Bernstein, J., & Ginsberg, S. (2009). Toward an integrated model of the scholarship of teaching and learning and faculty development. *Journal of Centers for Teaching and Learning, 1*, 41–55

Blackmore, J. A. (2005). A critical evaluation of peer review via teaching observation within higher education. *The International Journal of Educational Management, 19*(3), 218–232.

Blase, J., & Blase, J. (1999). *Leadership for staff development: Supporting the lifelong study of teaching and learning.* Retrieved from ERIC database (ED439123).

Burman, M. E., & Kleinsasser, A. (2004). Ethical guidelines for use of student work: Moving from teaching's invisibility to inquiry's visibility in the scholarship of teaching and learning. *The Journal of General Education, 53*(1), 59–79.

Carnegie Foundation for the Advancement of Teaching (2010). Basic Classification: Distribution of Institutions and Enrollments by Classification Category. *2010 Carnegie Classification.* Retrieved from http://classifications.carnegiefoundation.org/summary/basic.php

Christophel, D. M. (1990). The relationships among teacher immediacy behaviors, student motivation, and learning. *Communication Education, 39*, 323–340.

Council of Academic Programs in Communication Sciences and Disorders. (2009). *Report: 2009 CAPCSD survey of research doctoral students.* Retrieved from http://www.capcsd.org/documents/2009Doctoral SurveyResults.pdf

Darwin, A. & Palmer, E. (2009). Mentoring circles in higher education. *Higher Education Research & Development, 28*(2), 125-136.

Denzin, N. K., & Lincoln, Y. S. (2003). *Collecting and interpreting qualitative materials* (2nd ed.). Thousand Oaks, CA: Sage.

Eisner, E. W. (1998). *The enlightened eye: Qualitative inquiry and the enhancement of educational practice.* Upper Saddle River, NJ: Prentice Hall.

Esposito, J., & Smith, S. (2006). From reluctant teacher to empowered teacher-researcher: One educator's journey toward action research. *Teacher Education Quarterly, Summer,* 45–60.

Fink, L. D. (2003). *Creating significant learning experiences.* San Francisco, CA: Jossey-Bass.

Fischler, L. A., & Zachary, L. J. (2009). Shifting gears: The mentee in the driver's seat. *Adult Learning, 20*(1–2), 5–9.

Gardner, S. K. (2005). Faculty preparation for teaching, research, and service roles: What do new faculty need? *Journal of Faculty Development, 20*(3), 161–166.

Goodwin, L. D. (2004). A synergistic approach to faculty mentoring. *The Journal of Faculty Development, 19*(3), 145-152.

Hammersley-Fletcher, L., & Orsmond, P. (2004). Evaluating our peers: Is peer observation a meaningful process? *Studies in Higher Education, 29*(4), 489–503.

Hammersley-Fletcher, L., & Orsmond, P. (2005). Reflecting on reflective practices within peer observation. *Studies in Higher Education, 30*(2), 213–224.

Harland, T., & Plangger, G. (2004). The postgraduate chameleon: Changing roles in doctoral education. *Active Learning in Higher Education, 5*(1), 73–86

The Higher Education Academy. (2009). Peer observation of teaching. Oxford Brookes University: Oxford, UK. Retrieved from http://www.heacademy.ac.uk/hlst/resources/a-zdirectory/peer_observation

Hutchings, P. (2003). Competing goods: Ethical issues in the scholarship of teaching and learning. *Change, 35*(5), 26–33.

Hutchings, P. (2008, October). From special occasion to regular work. *Carnegie Perspectives*. Palo Alto, CA: The Carnegie Foundation. Retrieved from http://www.carnegiefoundation.org/perspectives/different-way-think-about-professional-development

Hutchings, P., & Shulman, L. S. (1999). The scholarship of teaching: New elaborations, new developments. *Change, Sept.–Oct.,* 11–15.

King, P., & Witt, P. (2009). Teacher immediacy, confidence testing, and the measurement of cognitive learning. *Communication Education, 58*(1), 110–123.

Lopez-Real, F., & Kwan, T. (2005). Mentors' perceptions of their own professional development during mentoring. *Journal of Education for Teaching, 31*(1), 15–24.

Maurer, T. W. (2011). On publishing SoTL articles. *International Journal for the Scholarship of Teaching and Learning, 5*(1). Retrieved from http://academics.georgiasouthern.edu/ijsotl/v5n1.html

McCormack, C., & West, D. (2006). Facilitated group mentoring develops key career competencies for university women: A case study. *Mentoring & Tutoring, 14*(4), 409–431.

McKinney, K. (2007). *Enhancing Learning Through the Scholarship of Teaching and Learning.* Boston, MA: Anker.

Nixom, S., Vickerman, P., & Maynard, C. (2010). Teacher immediacy: Reflections on a peer review of teaching scheme. *Journal of Further and Higher Education, 34*(4), 491–502.

Orjada, S. A., & Dachtyl, L. A. (2007, Spring). Approaching college teaching preparation in a scholarly manner: A tutorial. *Contemporary Issues in Communication Science and Disorders, 34,* 37–43.

Paulsen, M. B. (2001). The relationship between research and the scholarship of teaching. In C. Kreber (Ed.), *New Directions for teaching and learning: No. 86. Scholarship revisited: Perspectives on the scholarship of teaching* (pp. 19–29). San Francisco, CA: Jossey-Bass.

Postholm, M. B. (2008). Group work as a learning situation: A qualitative study in a university classroom. *Teachers and Teaching: Theory and Practice, 14*(2), 143–155.

Savage, II. E., Karp, R. S., & Logue, S. (2004). Faculty mentorship at colleges and universities. *College Teaching, 52*(1), 21–24.

Seidel, L. F., & Montgomery, B. (1996, June). *Formal academic programs in college teaching: A new model of preparing future faculty.* Paper presented at the National Center on Postsecondary Teaching, Learning, and Assessment. State College, PA.

Shortland, S. (2004). Peer observation: A tool for staff development or compliance? *Journal of Further and Higher Education, 28*(2), 219–228.

Shortland, S. (2010). Feedback within peer observation: Continuing professional development and unexpected consequences. *Innovations in Education and Teaching International, 47*(3), 295–304.

Shulman, L. S. (2004). *Teaching as community property.* San Francisco, CA: Jossey-Bass.

Smith, R. A. (2008). Moving toward the scholarship of teaching and learning: The classroom can be a lab too! *Teaching of Psychology, 35*(4), 262–266.

Tagg, J. (2011). What makes for a high quality SoTL research article? *International Journal for the Scholarship of Teaching and Learning, 5*(1). Retrieved from http://academics.georgiasouthern.edu/ijsotl/v5n1.html

Walstad, W. B., & Becker, W. E. (2010). Preparing graduate students in economics for teaching: Survey findings and recommendations. *The Journal of Economic Education, 41*(2), 202–210.

Weimer, M. (2008). Positioning scholarly work on teaching and learning. *International Journal for the Scholarship of Teaching and Learning, 2*(1). Retrieved from http://academics.georgiasouthern.edu/ijsotl/v5n1.html

Wineburg, S. S. (1991). On reading of historical texts: Notes on the breach between school and academy. *American Educational Research Journal, 28*(3), 495–519.

Zachary, L. J. (2002). The role of teacher as mentor. In J. M. Ross-Gordon (Ed.), *New directions for adult and continuing education: No. 93. Contemporary viewpoints on teaching adults effectively* (pp. 27–38). Wilmington, DE: Wiley Periodicals.

SOTL as Part of Your Research Agenda

> *It is possible to be teacher, practitioner and researcher all separately, but perhaps communication education is best served when these roles are blended with one another in mind.*
>
> —Seamon, 2005, p. 52

All faculty members should at the very least be involved in SOTL as consumers of SOTL research. However, it is your choice as to whether you want to be a producer of SOTL research. For faculty interested in participating in SOTL work within their discipline, this chapter outlines how to begin integrating classroom research into their research agenda and academic career. SOTL is not an easier type of research, but a different laboratory from which to study a research question. "The SoTL practitioner is at once a scholar of his or her own discipline *and* a scholar of learning and teaching within that discipline" (O'Brien, 2008, p. 1). SOTL requires the same "rigorous processes of research" (O'Brien, 2008, p. 1). Ludlow and Kent (2011) describe the characteristics of a successful scientist as including a love of science and curiosity, discipline and focus, flexible thinking, tolerance for failure and criticism, leadership skills, organizational skills, and networking skills. These are the same characteristics that an individual interested in conducting SOTL research must have;

however, the first characteristic could be reworded to be a love of and curiosity about teaching and learning. Pursuing SOTL research is not just about conducting research, but it is about becoming an expert teacher (Seamon, 2005) and maximizing student learning. As presented in Chapter 2, SOTL research is about the integration of pedagogical content knowledge (PCK) and teacher-learner interaction in making educational decisions in order to maximize student learning outcomes, and then making the research findings public.

Jumping right in to planning your SOTL research agenda may seem overwhelming. Maybe you are not at the point of actually doing your own SOTL research, or maybe you have the "fear of 'novice-stry'" (Tremonte, 2011). Novice-stry? According to Tremonte, novice-stry is when we "hesitate to undertake such work for fear and loathing of being novice again; of having to master new theories of and methodologies for investigating 'learning'" (p. 2). We already know our own discipline and how to conduct research in that area, so do we really want to begin to learn the discipline of teaching and learning? The answer is "yes" if you want to maximize your student learning outcomes.

But instead of jumping right in to doing your own SOTL research, you might need to develop or grow into it. As Chapter 1 presents, there is a continuum of educator development—starting with good teaching, then scholarly teaching, and progressing to SOTL. Weston and McAlpine (2001) propose a three-phase continuum of growth toward the scholarship of teaching. *Phase One: Growth in own teaching* begins by developing knowledge about your own teaching and about your students' learning. This is accomplished through activities such as, reading about teaching and learning, reflecting on the curriculum, reflecting on your own teaching and student learning within your classroom, and engaging in teaching development activities.

Phase Two: Dialogue with colleagues about teaching and learning—The goal is to increase your knowledge about teaching and learning within your discipline through engaging in conversations with colleagues (Weston & McAlpine, 2001). This phase includes conversations with colleagues about PCK; mentoring other teachers; becoming involved in teaching associations; organizing workshops within your department, division, or institution about teaching and learning; and increasing your knowledge and understanding about teaching and learning.

The final phase, *Phase Three: Growth in scholarship of teaching*, is focused on SOTL research (Weston & McAlpine, 2001). In this phase, you continue to develop your knowledge of SOTL with the goal of sharing your findings with your institution, colleagues, and others in the field. Phase three includes presenting and publishing SOTL research findings, mentorship of new or novice SOTL researchers, seeking funding for SOTL research, and expanding on your knowledge of SOTL.

Shulman (2004) identifies four kinds of scholars: successful pathfinders, successful pathfollowers, unsuccessful pathfinders and unsuccessful pathfollowers. Pathfollowers "behave as most of their disciplinary colleagues expect them to" (Shulman, 2004, p. vii), while pathfinders are "those who elect to go against the grain" (p. vii). To engage in SOTL research, we often must be the pathfinder who is going against the grain and not conforming to the disciplinary conventions; however, this means that we may also be going against the grain of the academic culture for our discipline (Vieira, 2009). This is particularly true on some campuses, while not on others. Therefore, it is critical that you know what is valued on your campus as you begin to plan your SOTL research agenda (discussed in Chapter 8).

Planning Your SOTL Research Agenda

Whether you are conducting basic, evidence-based research, clinical research, or SOTL research you need to have a plan. Francis (2007) lays out the basic elements or steps in getting started in SOTL research. His basic elements are as follows:

1. Identify the question, or describe what it is to be learned
2. Develop a plan to gather data
3. Gather and analyze data
4. Describe your results and generate a context for your results
5. State your conclusions
6. Share your results with peers (make your results public with an audience)
7. Make decisions about future action related to your question (p. 2).

As with any research, we must start with our research question or purpose of the project. For SOTL research, the question examines some aspect of teaching and its effect on student learning. Typically, the research question or purpose stems from experiences in the classroom and some issue, problem, concern, or challenge that is happening. The research question may come from your reflections on teaching and learning, discussions with other faculty members, and/or the literature or presentations on SOTL topics. The questions may focus on knowledge or skills that students are to acquire as a result of a course or activity; how students acquire specific knowledge; availability of or type of evidence that captures student learning; assessment tools or techniques that can be used to document learning; and so on (Smith, 2008). McKinney (2011) suggests examining gaps in the SOTL research in order to develop your research question. These gaps could include examining specific theories; co-curricular or extracurricular learning; graduate student learning; bottlenecks in learning; cross-disciplinary learning; cross-institutional aspects of teaching and learning; use of technology in the classroom; and methods of information delivery such as online, distance learning, and hybrid approaches, among others. Another way to determine your research questions is to tie them to institutional priorities, the institutional strategic plan, or other initiatives on your campus, such as the use of service learning, or undergraduate research (McKinney, 2011). Other research questions can stem from areas that we know are lacking research, such as information about the learner (i.e., what they know, believe, and expect and their framework of thinking), information about the faculty (i.e., what are their assumptions and expectations about the learner and teaching environment), unreliable areas of information (i.e., what happens for accreditation, use of student learning outcomes, and use of the course syllabi), and distorted information (i.e., credit hour—determines time in seat, but what about learning?; grades—distort students' perception of value of the experience; requirements—general education versus major) (Tagg, 2011).

Dewar (2008) proposes that SOTL research questions tend to fall into three areas. First are "What is?" questions, which attempt to describe a situation. For example, how does a communication sciences and disorders (CSD) majors' understanding of language disorders evolve as they move through the discipline? Or how do undergraduate CSD majors describe the fields of speech-language pathology and/or audiology? Or how do student descriptions compare to those of professionals in the field? A second category of questions are "What works?" These questions attempt to examine the effectiveness of specific pedagogical approaches, such as, determining which curricular offerings or clinical experiences have the most significant impact on the understanding of a specified clinical area; or examining whether a professional issues course encourages students to demonstrate appropriate professional behaviors in the clinical setting; or determining whether the demonstration of intervention approaches within the classroom setting leads to their appropriate use in the clinical setting. The final category of questions according to Dewar (2008) is "What could be?" questions. As the name implies, these questions connect the discipline to the real world. For example, how would students' perception of CSD be impacted if student were required to participate in service learning activities within all of their major courses?

After the research questions are identified, then the specific plan for how to answer the research question is developed. The research plan is based on PCK and knowledge about the teacher-learner interaction. In devising your SOTL research plan, we would suggest considering Weimer's (2006) classification of scholarly work (discussed in Chapter 2), as this may provide you with ideas as to the type of scholarly work you are planning. We also recommend that you consider the level of evidence that the SOTL research will be providing (also in Chapter 2). For example, will the study provide lower levels of evidence in the form of wisdom-of-practice through personal accounts of change, recommended practice reports, recommended-content reports, or personal narratives; or will it be a qualitative or descriptive study; or the highest level of evidence available in the form of a quantitative investigation? As with any research plan, your SOTL research plan should be specific as to what data will be collected, how it will be collected, and how the data will be analyzed in order to answer the research question(s) being posed.

After the plan has been developed and IRB approval has been obtained (see Chapter 8), then the SOTL researcher is ready to conduct the study and analyze and interpret the results. However, at this point the results are only impacting your own classroom, and the findings are not scholarship until they are made public so that others can build on our work. Therefore, the results need to not only be shared with the colleagues within your department, division, college, and institution, but also beyond the walls of your institution. This critical review of your work will enable you to receive feedback, which will help you to make decisions about the future direction of your SOTL research. In addition, it will enable others to build on the work that you have done. Disseminating your findings is a critical step in moving your research from scholarly teaching to the SOTL.

The Value of SOTL on Your Campus?

Variability by Type of Institution

As you embark on developing your SOTL research plan, make sure that you know whether SOTL is valued on your campus. Does your promotion and tenure system view SOTL as counting for scholarship? Or does only discipline specific scholarship count? If you are not sure of the answers for these questions, then it is vital that you find it out so as to not commit career suicide.

As Chapter 8 points out, there are several ways to find out whether SOTL is valued on your campus. However, just because SOTL is valued on a campus, does not mean that it is counted as scholarship when it comes to the promotion and tenure process. Although SOTL research is being included and is counting in the promotion and tenure process at more institutions, do not just assume that it will count (Weimer, 2006). We strongly recommend that you find out whether SOTL research counts as scholarship for the promotion and tenure process that you will be or are a part of. To do so, we recommend that you start by talking to your department chairperson, academic dean, colleagues, and, if you have a center for teaching and learning, talking to the director. These individuals should be able to provide you with insight as to the value of SOTL in this process.

Utilizing the Carnegie Classification System, there are three general types of institutions of higher education where CSD programs tend to be found: research institutions, comprehensive institutions, and liberal arts institutions. Research institutions offer a wide range of undergraduate programs and are committed to graduate education through the doctorate level. If you are employed at a research institution, then chances are that scholarship only means discipline-specific scholarship and not SOTL research. Thus, the chances are slim that SOTL research would carry any weight in your application for promotion or tenure.

Comprehensive institutions offer a wide range of undergraduate programs and have graduate programs through the master's level. The definition of scholarship will vary at these institutions. Some of the comprehensive institutions will define research as discipline specific research, while others will include SOTL research. Therefore, you really need to determine what is expected with regards to scholarship.

The third general type of institution is the liberal arts college, whose primary emphasis is on undergraduate education. For the most part, these institutions tend to have academic cultures that not only emphasize excellence in teaching, but also encourage SOTL research. The liberal arts institutions tend to have more flexible promotion and tenure guidelines with regards to research; thus, scholarship is thought of broadly and includes both traditional discipline-specific research, as well as SOTL research.

Regardless of the type of academic institution that you are employed at or are seeking employment at, you need to remember that there are differences both between and within institution types. Thus, we highly recommend that you find out what the expectations are on your specific campus as you plan your research agenda and the role that SOTL will play.

Why the Variability within and between Institutions?

Aside from the type of institution, the promotion and tenure process varies from one campus to the next and SOTL counts on some campuses and not others for many possible reasons. One of the possible reasons is that many institutions do not have any formal definition of SOTL (McKinney, 2007). The lack of a formal definition or even recognition of SOTL as a scholarly activity can lead to institutions that do not value SOTL in their promotion and tenure process. Definitions allow for a standard manner of viewing and discussing SOTL. Institutions that have a clearly stated definition or mission with regards to SOTL provide their faculty with a way to classify the work that they are doing. In addition, institutions with clear definitions and recognition of the value of SOTL tend to also reward SOTL activities in the promotion and tenure process. However, even those institutions with statements regarding to SOTL can demonstrate variability due to the difficulty in defining SOTL, as well as variability in the expectations of departments and programs. As Boshier (2009) states "scholarship of teaching is used as a synonym for other activities" (p. 1), and this leads to confusion by the faculty and administration. This confusion stems from "conceptual confusion" (Boshier, 2009, p. 1) of Boyer's (1990) definition of scholarship (see Chapter 1).

Changing expectations by rotating department chairs and/or committee members is another reason for the variability across and within institutions. As our definitions or interpretation of the definition of SOTL changes from institution to institution and from one individual to the next, it makes it difficult for faculty members to know what to expect. For example, the junior faculty member meets with the department chair when they are first hired. Together, they create a plan for scholarship which includes SOTL research in their research agenda; however, as time progresses and the faculty member implements their plan, the department chair changes, and they hit a bump in the road. The new department chair interprets the definition of SOTL differently and does not view SOTL as scholarly work that counts towards promotion and/or tenure. Or the bump in the road may be in the form of the composition of the promotion and tenure committee and their view of scholarship. It, thus, appears to the faculty member seeking promotion or tenure that the performance expectations are inconsistent and shifting (Sorcinelli, 2002). This ambiguity due to the rotation of chairs and committee members leads to a flawed review system and tension between the ideal system on paper and the reality faced by faculty members (Sorcinelli, 2002).

What Can Be Done?

Changing the Value of SOTL on Your Campus

So, if there is such variability within and between institutions, what can faculty members do? We believe that we need to change the value of SOTL on campuses, so that it has the same value as discipline-specific research. When we look at our responsibilities as faculty members, previous research has found that most of us spend at least 40% of our time in teaching related activities, 40% on research, and the remaining 20% on administrative and service-related activities (Knapper, 1997). However, the majority of us do not work at research institutions, which means that we work at institutions where teaching is an even larger percentage of our responsibilities or where teaching and research are intertwined and not distinct and competing job responsibilities (Marincovich, 2007; Tinberg, Duffy, & Mino, 2007). Therefore, if teaching is the major portion of our job, or intertwined with our research, then why is it not valued more? How can we change the value that our institutions place on teaching and SOTL?

One of the ways that we as faculty members can help to change the value of SOTL at our institutions is to initiate conversations with colleagues on campus about SOTL. The conversation can start at the departmental or programmatic level with something as basic as having faculty members agree on learning outcomes for courses and a protocol for measuring whether the outcomes have been met or not (Wieman, 2007). Another way to start the conversation within CSD programs is to advocate for the use and value of evidence-based education (EBE) and comparing it to the use and value of evidence-based practice (EBP) in the clinical setting. Starting the dialogue with colleagues is like throwing a pebble in a still pond. It will start to ripple and spread throughout the pond, throughout the institution. As McKinney (2011) stated "people aren't opposed to SOTL; they are just oblivious to it." Therefore, we must start the conversation and get the ripple flowing through our institutions. If you are a junior-level faculty member and worried about starting this conversation for fear of it having a negative impact on your future at the institution, then we would recommend encouraging trusted tenured faculty to initiate the conversation. If you still cannot get the conversation rippling at your own institution, then have conversations about SOTL with colleagues at other institutions. These conversations, whether within the institution or between colleagues at different institutions, can focus on examining current SOTL research, student learning within a specific discipline, pedagogical approaches and their impact on student learning, advocacy of SOTL and EBE, among others.

In addition to starting the dialogue, it is important to get college/university administrators to value and support SOTL (Hoessler, Britnell, & Stockley, 2010). Administrative support of SOTL is critical. In addition to administrators recruiting, hiring, and promoting excellent teachers (Umbach, 2007), they can support SOTL in many forms including the following: developing an institutional statement on the value of SOTL, defining categories of teaching and learning activities, expanding the range of scholarly activities that are rewarded by the institution, and/or the creation or support of a center for teaching and learning. It could also be done by examining the "SOTL accomplishments, practices, and activities . . . of the individual, the discipline, organizational unit" (Quinnell, Russell, Thompson, Marshall, & Cowley, 2010, p. 27), which increases the visibility of SOTL and sustains SOTL practices within the group. If the administration is truly going to support SOTL, then there also needs to be some funding for SOTL research on the campus. Even small stipends, grants, and/or release time can help to support faculty members who are conducting SOTL research and encourage faculty members to become involved in SOTL research.

Furthermore, conversations should also focus on how SOTL is a "legitimate form of scholarship" (Smith, 2008, p. 262) that should be rewarded in annual reviews and the promotion and tenure process. These discussions can include the argument that SOTL is based on theory and previous research. It is planned research that has IRB approval and leads to the collection of objective data from which practices and conclusions are drawn (Wieman, 2007), and original knowledge is developed. In addition, as has been mentioned throughout this book, the findings must be made public for others to review, challenge, and build upon in order for it to be SOTL research; otherwise it is just scholarly teaching.

By changing the value of SOTL at an institution, it will also benefit the institution. For example, SOTL can provide an avenue for strengthening faculty development efforts on a campus (Dewar, 2008; Sorcinelli, Austin, Eddy, & Beach, 2006). It can enable an institution to examine priority teaching issues (i.e., undergraduate research, study abroad, service learning) and demonstrate their impact on learning, retention, and student engagement. SOTL research can examine strategic planning initiatives, which benefits the institution. It can strengthen the connections between clinical and academic faculty members and/or between faculty members of different disciplines.

As you examine and develop an approach to changing the value of SOTL on your campus, remember that no single approach is going to work. It is going to take many approaches over a long period of time that will hopefully lead to a change in the institutional culture and the value of SOTL (Ginsberg & Bernstein, 2011). So be patient. Start small and keep moving forward.

Changing the Value of SOTL Within CSD

In addition to changing the value of SOTL at the institutional level, we also need to make changes within our state, regional, and national associations. Changes are beginning to occur at the national level within the American Speech-Language-Hearing Association (ASHA). For many years there has been the Special Interest Group (SIG) (previously known as Special Interest Division) 10: Issues in Higher Education. SIG 10 has championed the broad issues faced within higher education, and in the more recent years, it has addressed the importance of SOTL within the fields of CSD. For the very first time, the 2011 ASHA convention presented a topic area for SOTL in CSD, which was separate from the Academic and Educational Issues topic area. This provided members with short courses, seminars, and poster presentations regarding SOTL. The future hope would be that professional publications dedicated to SOTL in CSD would also be developed. It is critical that ASHA, as well as other national organizations, and their membership not only learn about SOTL, but that they come to value SOTL in CSD as we educate future professionals.

Final Thoughts

When we set off to write a book about SOTL in CSD fields, we did so with the hope that it would lead to others seeing the value of SOTL for the field. We did so with the hope of sharing what we have learned about SOTL in order to make a difference in the lives of our students. In the end what really matters is not whether SOTL counts for promotion and tenure or that it is valued by our institutions or associations, but rather that by participating in SOTL research, we incorporated pedagogical approaches that are based on evidence, that lead to improved learning in our students, and enrich both the lives of our students, our communities, and ourselves. It is important that SOTL be a part of CSD. It will make a difference, which after all, is the reason why the vast majority of us chose to work in the fields of CSD. Our challenge to you is to take that first step, toss the pebble, and incorporate SOTL in your CSD work.

References

Boyer, E. L. (1990). *Scholarship reconsidered: Priorities of the professoriate*. San Francisco, CA: Jossey-Bass.

Boshier, R. (2009). Why is the scholarship of teaching and learning such a hard sell? *Higher Education Research & Development, 28*(1), 1–15. doi: 10.1080/07294360802444321

Dewar, J. M. (2008). An apology for the scholarship of teaching and learning. *InSight: A Journal of Scholarly Teaching, 3*, 17–22.

Francis, R. (2007). Getting started with SoTL in your classroom. *International Journal for the Scholarship of Teaching and Learning, 1*(2), 1–4. Retrieved from http://www.georgiasouthern.edu/ijsotl

Ginsberg, S. M., & Bernstein, J. L. (2011). Growing the scholarship of teaching and learning through institutional culture change. *Journal of the Scholarship of Teaching and Learning, 11*(1), 1–12.

Hoessler, C., Britnell, J., & Stockley, D. (2010). Assessing the impact of educational development through the lens of the scholarship of teaching and learning. *New Directions for Teaching and Learning, 122*, 81–89.

Knapper, C. (1997). Rewards for teaching. *New Directions for Teaching and Learning, 72*, 41–52.

Ludlow, C. L., & Kent, R. D. (2011). *Building a research career.* San Diego, CA: Plural.

Marincovich, M. (2007). Teaching and learning in a research-intensive university. In R. P. Perry & J. C. Smart (Eds.), *The scholarship of teaching and learning in higher education: An evidence-based perspective* (pp. 23–37). The Netherlands: Springer.

McKinney, K. (2007). *Enhancing learning through the scholarship of teaching and learning: The challenges and joys of juggling.* San Francisco, CA: Anker.

McKinney, K. (2011). *Making a difference: Application of SOTL beyond the classroom to enhancing learning.* Keynote presentation at the SOTL Academy, Eastern Michigan University, Ypsilanti, MI.

O'Brien, M. (2008). Navigating the SoTL landscape: A compass, map and some tools for getting started. *International Journal for the Scholarship of Teaching and Learning, 2*(2), 1–20. Retrieved from http://www.goergiasouthern.edu/ijsotl

Quinnell, R., Russell, C., Thompson, R., Marshall, N., & Cowley, J. (2010). Evidence-based narratives to reconcile teaching practices in academic discipline with the scholarship of teaching and learning. *Journal of the Scholarship of Teaching and Learning, 10*(3), 20–30.

Seamon, M. (2005). The communication triad: A participatory model for the scholarship of teaching and learning in communication. *Journal of Scholarship of Teaching and Learning, 5*(1), 46–53.

Shulman, L. S. (2004). Four-word: Against the Grain. In M. Huber (Ed.), *Balancing acts: The scholarship of teaching and learning in academic careers.* Retrieved from http://www.carnegiefoundation.org/sites/default/files/Balancing_acts_Four-word.pdf

Smith, R. A. (2008). Moving toward the scholarship of teaching and learning: The classroom can be a lab, too! *Teaching of Psychology, 35*, 262–266. doi: 10.1080/00986280802418711

Sorcinelli, M. D. (2002). New conceptions of scholarship for new generation of faculty members. *New Directions for Teaching and Learning, 90*, 41–47.

Sorcinelli, M. D., Austin, A. E., Eddy, P. L., & Beach, A. L. (2006). *Creating the future faculty development: Learning from the past, understanding the present.* Bolton, MA: Anker.

Tagg, J. (2011). *Using SoTL to dispel the fog of learning.* Keynote presentation at the SOTL Academy, Eastern Michigan University, Ypsilanti, MI.

Tinberg, H., Duffy, D. K., & Mino, J. (2007). The scholarship of teaching and learning at the two-year college: Promise and peril. *Change,* 26–33. Retrieved from http://www.changemag.org/Archives/Back%20Issues/July-August%202008/full-listening-to-students.html

Tremonte, C. M. (2011). Window shopping: Fashioning a scholarship of interdisciplinary teaching and learning. *International Journal for Scholarship of Teaching and Learning, 5*(1), 1–9. Retrieved from http://www.georgiasouthern.edu/ijsotl

Umbach, P. D. (2007). Faculty cultures and college teaching. In R. P. Perry and J. C. Smart (Eds.), *The scholarship of teaching and learning in higher education: An evidence-based perspective* (pp. 263–317). The Netherlands: Springer.

Vieira, F. (2009). Developing the scholarship of pedagogy: Pathfinding in adverse settings. *Journal of the Scholarship of Teaching and Learning, 9*(2), 10–21.

Weimer, M. (2006). *Enhancing scholarly work on teaching and learning: Professional literature that makes a difference.* San Francisco, CA: Jossey-Bass.

Weston, C. B., & McApline, L. (2001). Making explicit the development toward the scholarship of teaching. *New Directions for Teaching and Learning, 86,* 89–97.

Wieman, C. (2007). Why not try a scientific approach to science education. *Change.* Retrieved from http://www.changemag.org/Archives/Back Issues/September-October 2007/full-scientific-approach.html

Index

A

Academic service learning (ASL), 142–150. *See also* Service learning
Active learning, 42, 48–51, 146
Assessment, 60, 72–73, 169–195. *See also* Feedback
  academic prompts, 60
  authentic assessment, 175–179, 182
  course evaluation, 15, 156
  criteria and standards, 72, 73
  evidence-based assessment, 170, 182
  FIDeLity feedback, 72, 73
  formative, 10, 61, 172–175, 177–179, 182–189
  informal checks of understanding, 60–61
  mid-term feedback, 15–17
  performance tasks, 60, 66
  quiz and test items, 60
  self-assessment, 63, 72, 73, 182
  summative, 10, 162, 171–172, 173, 175, 176–179, 208

B

Backward design, 58–67, 69
  evidence for, 64–65
  six facets of understanding, 59, 65
  stages of, 58–64
  WHERETO, 62–64
Bloom's Taxonomy, 42–46, 51, 59, 65, 67
Boyer, Ernest, 1–3, 33, 244

C

Carnegie classification system, 200–202, 243
Carroll, John, 10
Centers for teaching and learning. *See* Teaching and learning centers (TLC)
Classroom climate, 130–133
Civic
  awareness, 142
  engagement, 147
Clarity 109–111
  teacher clarity short inventory, 110
Classroom assessment techniques (CATs), 188–193
  applications cards, 190–191, 193
  everyday ethical dilemmas, 191, 193
  minute paper, 61, 85, 189–190, 192
  muddiest point, 190, 192
  one sentence summary, 190, 193
Clickers, 156–160. *See also* Electronic student response system and Personal response systems

251

Collaborative learning techniques (CLTs), 128–136
Community Building Activities (CBA), 115–117
Community service, 142, 144
Constructivism, 48
 constructivist teaching, 48, 137

D

Doctoral program support, 200–202

E

Educator development, 9, 11–13, 22, 203, 238
Electronic student response systems, 156. *See also* Clickers and Personal response systems
Evidence-based education (EBE), 18–19, 28–30, 35, 41, 57, 69, 170, 197, 245
 definition, 28–30
 finding evidence, 38
 levels of evidence, 30–35
 model, 29
 need for, 36–37
 research scholarship, 31–32
 wisdom-of-practice, 31, 32–34
Evidence-based practice (EBP), 25–28, 35, 245
 definition, 25
 levels of evidence, 27–28, 35
 model, 26
 types of evidence, 26

F

Faculty learning communities, 18–22
Family Educational Rights and Privacy Act (FERPA), 224
Feedback
 communication 98–99, 132
 course design, use in, 64–65
 feedback and assessment, 72–75, 172–174, 179. *See also* Assessment in situ feedback 156–159
 from peer observations, 207–211, 232. *See also* Peer Observation of Teaching (POT) regarding SOTL studies, 229–230
Fink, L. Dee, 7, 45–46, 64–79, 84–90

G

Good teaching, 9–10, 13, 17

H

Humanistic teachers, 112

I

Immediacy, 100–108, 111–112, 119–121
 immediacy behaviors, 102–103
In-class discussions, 129–133
Instructional communication competence, 98–100
Internet-based teaching, 151–153
Interpersonal relationships, 100

K

Knowledge and skills acquisition (KASA), 33, 58, 68, 73

L

Learner centered instruction, 47–53, 98

M

Mentoring, 203–207, 238
  active mentorship, 147
  effective mentors, 207
  group mentoring, 205
  mentoring circles, 205
  synergistic mentoring, 204

O

Observation
  informal peer, 17
  Peer Observation of Teaching (POT), 207–211
Online communication
  asynchronous discussion, 153, 160, 163
  etiquette, 118
  synchronous communication, 117

P

Pedagogical content knowledge (PCK), 4, 5, 29, 30, 33, 37, 38, 46 69, 229, 238, 241
Peer teaching, 52, 87, 133–136
Personal response systems, 156. *See also* Clickers and Electronic student response systems
Philosophy of teaching, 112–113
Podcasting, 153–155, 162–163
Preparing Future Faculty 6
Problem-based learning (PBL), 119, 137–141, 222–223, 228

Promotion and tenure, 15, 36, 80, 198, 206, 208, 229, 230, 242, 243, 244, 246, 248

R

Rapport talk, 100
Research
  action research, 211–218
  collaboration with students, 225–226
  ethical considerations, 217–226
  institutional review board approval, 221, 224–226, 227, 228, 241, 246
  public dissemination, 11, 20, 21, 154, 214, 226, 229–232
  qualitative, 31–32, 34, 35, 86, 88, 99, 213–215, 217, 225, 231
  quantitative, 31, 34, 35, 65, 85, 87, 88, 213, 214, 215, 231
Reflective thinking. 9, 48, 51–53, 139, 144, 146. *See also* Student reflection
Rubrics, 182–188
  analytic rubrics, 180, 183, 184
  holistic rubrics, 183, 186

S

Scholarly teaching, 9, 10, 13, 18
Scholarship
  of application, 2, 33
  of discovery, 1, 2, 3, 4
  of integration, 2, 3, 33
  teaching, 2–3
Scholarship of teaching and learning (SOTL), 28, 37, 38, 57
  changing the value on campus, 244–247
  four kinds of scholars, 239

Scholarship of teaching and learning (SOTL) *(continued)*
 research agenda or research plan, 239–242,
 research questions, 240
 sources of research, 38
 value with CSD, 247
 variability between institutions, 242–244
Shulman, Lee, 3, 4, 5, 10, 29, 33, 239,
Self-disclosures, 112–114
Service learning, 240, 241, 247. *See also* Academic service learning
 direct service learning, 143–144
 indirect service learning, 143–144
Significant learning, 7
 application, 68, 70
 caring, 68, 71
 creating, 58, 64, 65–91
 evidence for, 85–88
 foundational knowledge, 68, 70
 grading system, 78
 human dimension, 68, 70–71
 integration, 68, 70
 learning how to learn, 68, 71–72
 six interacting dimensions of learning, 65, 68, 69–72
Social networking, 117–118, 121
Social presence, 114–121
STOLEN Principle, 161–162
Student motivation, 15, 99, 115

Student reflection, 51–53, 146. *See also* Reflective thinking
Syllabus, 79–84, 106, 119, 155, 162, 179, 223

T

Teacher caring, 112
Teacher-learner interaction, 29, 30, 31, 37, 38, 68, 69, 238, 241
Teaching and learning centers (TLC), 8, 15–16,18, 20–21, 199, 202–203, 208, 209, 220, 230, 231, 232, 242, 246
Teaching strategy, 76–77, 129, 137, 138, 159
Teaching technique, 76–77, 138
Teacher transparency, 111–114
Technology-based learning, 148–163

U

University mission, 198, 244

W

Weimer, M., 31, 32, 33, 241, 242, 250
Wikis, 160–162

V

Volunteerism, 142